PRAISE FOR

GOING THE DISTANCE

"For a long time, I have felt a list of practical suggestions that should be provided would be valuable to runners. Paul Greer's experiences as an elite runner and a coach to varied levels of talent qualifies him as the perfect person to write this book. *Going the Distance* is full of concise, plainly stated information that is essential for distance runners to reach their full potential. I will keep a copy handy to refer to time and time again."

—Bob Larsen,
Four-time NCAA Coach of the Year while at UCLA, 2004 Olympic Distance Coach, National Track & Field Hall of Fame, USATF Legend Coach

"*Going the Distance* is full of useful information for runners at all levels. I would highly recommend Coach Paul Greer's book to prepare for a half or full marathon. His knowledge from his decade's long work with the San Diego Track Club is shared so others can learn from what Coach Paul Greer has discovered. This book is full of small tips that can provide huge rewards if you apply them to your routine. So, don't wait any longer and buy my friend's new book, *Going the Distance.*"

—Meb Keflezighi,
Four-time Olympian, 2004 Olympic Marathon Silver Medalist, 2009 New York Marathon Champion & 2014 Boston Marathon Champion

"Paul Greer came from elite runner to training people at all levels — from beginners anxious to run their first half-marathon to more seasoned competitors. Not only is Paul a knowledgeable coach, he is also a tremendous motivator! This book will get you off the couch and train for your new personal best!"

—Steve Scott
Three-time Olympian (1980, 1984, 1988)
Has run the most sub-four-minute miles in history at 136

"Coach Paul Greer led the team of supporters who had the vision to commemorate the 50th anniversary of my first sub-four-minute mile on June 5, 2014. Not only have Paul and his wife Callie become dear friends, Paul is a leader who lives what he teaches/coaches. (His love for the Lord affects each individual he comes in contact with, encouraging warmth and enthusiasm.) *Going the Distance* is a fantastically informative book filled with over 250 fitness/running tips that will help you reach your fullest potential. This book is for everyone who desires to maintain (or start) a good mental and physical health plan for their lives."

—Jim Ryun
Three-time Olympian (1964, 1968, 1972)
1968 Olympic 1500 Meter Silver Medalist,
Former World Record Holder (1 Mile, 1500m, 880 yards, 800m)
Recipient of the Presidential Medal of Freedom, July 2020

GOING
THE
DISTANCE

STRATEGIES FROM THE FIRST STRIDE
TO THE FINISH LINE

PAUL GREER

ACORN
PUBLISHING

FROM THE TINY ACORN …
GROWS THE MIGHTY OAK

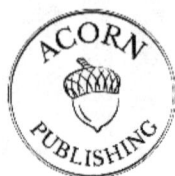

WWW.ACORNPUBLISHINGLLC.COM

For information, address:
Acorn Publishing, LLC
3943 Irvine Blvd. Ste. 218
Irvine, CA 92602

Going the Distance

Edited by Michele Wallace
Cover design by Damonza
All photography by Craig Kerstetter
Interior design and formatting by Jessica Therrien

Printed in the United States of America

ISBN-13: 979-8-88528-043-3 (hardcover)
ISBN-13: 979-8-88528-042-6 (paperback)
LCCN #: 2023915289

DEDICATED TO MY SUPPORT TEAM

Coach Dan Schaitel

Coach Jerry Downey

Coach Mike Healy

Coach Jim Cerveny

Coach Dixon Farmer

Coach Tom Lux

Coach Rahn Scheffield

Steve Scott

My Sister Michelle

My Dad

My Wife Callie

The countless teammates, training partners and friends who have made a difference in my life.

INTRODUCTION

Paul Greer has been a professor in Health and Exercise Science at San Diego City College for the past thirty-four years and has a master's degree in Kinesiology from Azusa Pacific University. Paul is a well-known staple amongst the San Diego running community, having coached thousands of athletes in endurance sports, including mid-distance track athletes, marathon runners, Ironman triathletes, and various endurance sport enthusiasts. His athletes include hundreds of Boston qualifiers, several top age-group competitors, and a handful of Olympic qualifiers.

One of the founding fathers of the San Diego Track Club, Paul has been a SDTC coach for nearly forty years. Paul also serves as the Director for the "Rockin N Runnin" full and half marathon training program. In 2016, Paul was selected to be the Men's Coach for Team USA's Senior (20-35) and Junior's teams (19 and under) at the Great Edinburgh Cross Country Championships. Paul has been a regular contributor in the past for SignOnSanDiego and San Diego Newsroom.

Before Paul started coaching, he was a very successful runner himself. A top San Diego section miler at St. Augustine High School, Paul was inducted into the school's Hall of Fame in 1995. After high school he went on to become the school record-holder for 1500 meters at San Diego State. His 3:42.44 still stands as the best mark in school history. Greer also ran the mile in under four minutes (3:59.79), was a 1992 U.S. Olympic Trials qualifier at 1500 meters with a 3:39.05, and competed in the tough European track circuit as a post collegian.

But Paul's resume isn't what is most impressive. Rather, it is Paul's sincere passion to improve lives through the pursuit of mental and physical excellence. Paul recognizes that every athlete has a story, and he enjoys

I

encouraging his athletes every step of the way . . . from the first stride in a pair of running shoes, through the celebrated finish line.

The running and fitness tips provided in this book cater to runners of all ages and abilities. These helpful tips will undoubtedly help you to reach your full potential and achieve your fitness goals.

HOW TO APPROACH THIS BOOK FOR MAXIMUM BENEFITS

Mankind has been running for centuries. In prehistoric times, we ran for survival. In today's modern world, we run for fitness, competition, and achievement. The knowledge you will gain by reading this book will help you reach your full potential.

This book provides one fitness tip per page. When reading, you can approach it in one of two ways:

Read the entire book in chronological order from the beginning to the end and learn about all aspects of running,

-or-

Review the book's table of contents and turn to the specific fitness tips that interest you, including:

- Tips for beginning a running program
- Breathing tips
- Nutrition tips
- Hydration tips
- Tips for taking your workouts to the next level
- Tips on training for a race
- Race day performance tips
- Tips for prevention and treatment of common ailments

READY. SET. GO!

As you look towards your running and fitness future, the knowledge and tips contained in *Going the Distance* will transform how you think about your training. You will have the knowledge to elevate your running to the next level.

Through your continued hard work and perseverance, your fitness and running goals will be achieved!

"You do not have to be asleep to have a dream!"

—Paul Greer
Professor, Health and Exercise Science, San Diego City College
San Diego Track Club Coach
Sub-Four Minute Miler (3:59.79)

Disclaimer: No copyright infringement is intended. I do not own, nor claim to own, any of the original fitness tips used in this book. This book contains facts combined with my real-world coaching and running experiences. *Going the Distance* is designed for educational purposes only, and its purpose is not to give medical advice or professional services. The information provided in this book should not be used for diagnosing or treating health and/or fitness concerns and/or disease. It is not a substitute for professional care. If you have, or suspect you may have, a health concern you should consult your healthcare provider.

TABLE OF CONTENTS

NUTRITION TIPS

HYDRATION TIPS

TIPS FOR TAKING YOUR WORKOUTS TO THE NEXT LEVEL

TIPS ON TRAINING FOR A RACE

RACE DAY PERFORMANCE TIPS

TIPS FOR PREVENTION & TREATMENT OF COMMON AILMENTS

WHAT I'VE LEARNED

"*Some people create with words or with music or with a brush and paints. I like to make something beautiful when I run.*"

– Steve Prefontaine

TIPS FOR BEGINNING A RUNNING PROGRAM

THE BENEFITS OF EXERCISE

In my humble opinion, there are two callings in life that will lead us to achieve our full potential as human beings. First is to love — love fearlessly and without limitation. Second is to share that love with others through our unique gifts and talents.

To accomplish this, we need to maintain good health, which requires us to focus on our own individualized health and exercise. While no amount of exercise can guarantee longevity, moderate amounts of exercise can improve the likelihood of a healthy life. Along with a positive attitude and a healthy diet, your fitness level plays a major role in how well you feel and the quality of life you enjoy.

Below are twelve benefits of fitness that I often share with my San Diego City College students and San Diego Track Club runners:

BENEFITS OF FITNESS

1. Relieves tension and stress
2. Provides enjoyment and fun
3. Stimulates the mind
4. Helps maintain stable weight
5. Controls appetite
6. Boosts self-image
7. Improves muscle tone and strength
8. Improves flexibility
9. Lowers blood pressure
10. Relieves insomnia
11. Increases good (HDL) cholesterol
12. Prevents diabetes

BARRIERS TO EXERCISE

Most people will agree exercise is good for you when done correctly; however, the fact remains that only 23 percent of the US population engage in exercise three or more days of the week. Over the years I have found when associating with other fitness enthusiasts that there are six barriers to exercise that are all easy to overcome:

1. **No Time?** Try shorter periods of activity spread throughout the day such as two twenty-minute runs.

2. **Too Tired?** It's often a lack of exercise that makes you feel tired. Exercise gives you energy.

3. **Embarrassed?** Be proud of the fact that you're taking care of your body.

4. **No Training Partner?** It's fun to exercise with others; however, if your regular partner quits then find another one. You are also free to join a fitness club, take a class, or exercise to a video.

5. **Bad Weather?** Too hot, cold, wet, or windy — it never seems right for exercise. Lots of people exercise come rain or shine. Try a variety of indoor and outdoor activities.

6. **Too Costly?** Try a low-cost option such as running instead of driving.

BEGINNERS RUNNING QUESTIONS

I oversee group workouts every Tuesday, and throughout the years I have been asked specific questions on how to get started in a running program. Below are five of the more common questions that I address with beginners regarding running:

HOW DO I START RUNNING?

My suggestion is you start walking for a period that feels comfortable, which can be anywhere from ten to thirty minutes. Once you can walk for thirty minutes easily, proceed and add one to two-minute running sessions into your walking. As time goes on, make the running sessions longer, until you're running for a solid thirty minutes.

SHOULD I BREATHE THROUGH MY NOSE OR MY MOUTH?

I suggest you do both. It's normal and natural to breathe through your nose and mouth at the same time. It's good to keep your mouth slightly open and relax your jaw muscles.

I ALWAYS FEEL OUT OF BREATH WHEN I RUN. IS SOME-THING WRONG?

Yes, you're probably trying to run too fast so relax and slow down. One of the fundamental mistakes a beginner can make is to run too fast. Concentrate on breathing from deep down in your abdomen and when necessary, take walking breaks.

I OFTEN SUFFER FROM A SIDE CRAMP WHEN I RUN. HOW DOES IT GO AWAY?

Unfortunately, side stitches are more common among beginners because your abdomen is not used to the movement that running causes. In my experience most runners find that stitches go away as fitness increases. I also suggest you try not to eat any solid foods during the hour before you run. When you get a stitch, breathe deeply, concentrating on pushing all the air out of your abdomen. By doing this it will stretch out your diaphragm muscle, which is usually where a cramp occurs.

IS IT NORMAL TO FEEL PAIN DURING RUNNING?

I believe discomfort is normal as you add distance and intensity to your training. However, real pain is not normal. If part of your body feels so bad that you run with a limp or otherwise alter your stride, you have a problem. Immediately stop running and take a few days off. If you are unsure about the pain, try walking for a minute or two to see if the discomfort disappears.

Remember to give yourself time to improve. Be patient, grow stronger, get faster, and run like the wind!

TIPS FOR RUNNING

During the 38 years coaching the San Diego Track Club many people have approached me who are taking up the sport of running for the first time. Below are a few guidelines to follow as you begin and continue with the lifelong activity of running.

Keep in mind that everyone improves at a different rate and some people can jog for an hour after four weeks, others take four months or a year to reach that point. Don't get discouraged. Continue to work at your aerobic level and listen to your own body. Eventually you will get there.

Your reward from running done gradually, comfortably, and pleasantly will be a new life. You will look and feel better physically and mentally.

- Think of running and exercise in terms of frequency not intensity, pleasure not pain. Use it as a reward to yourself.
- In warm weather, run early in the mornings or evenings.
- Exercise is cumulative so look for the long-term results.
- Vary your running periodically and this will keep running a fresh experience.
- Finally, think positive thoughts and you will improve.

TWO TRAINING MISTAKES YOU WANT TO AVOID

There are two training mistakes that I have observed athletes make over the years and especially those times when runners are preparing for longer distances including the marathon and half marathon.

1. Do not ignore your recovery days when training. They should be active recovery, meaning you can participate in some type of activity — if it's not running. I recommend taking one to two days off a week from running but not from exercising. Active recovery means you should be swimming, cycling, or engaging in another activity you enjoy on your day off. This is the time for you to rest and relax both mentally and physically from running. You should not overlook the importance of the time your body needs to recover from and adapt to the stresses of hard running.

2. Always remember to keep yourself fully hydrated no matter the time of year. Too often runners will forget to drink, particularly during the winter months when they might not be sweating as heavily. Do not allow yourself to become chronically dehydrated; it will severely compromise your health along with your training. I recommend you drink between 80 and 120 ounces of water daily.

REST AND RECOVERY IS CRITICALLY IMPORTANT

Rest and recovery can be the forgotten training principle. From my standpoint, recovery run days are the second most important day for everyone who participates in a full and half marathon training program. Most training adaptations occur during recovery, which is why it is such a vital component to an athlete's training.

As an athlete accumulates more years of training experience, less recovery time is needed because the body becomes more resilient underneath the current stimuli. Research has shown than an individual needs a minimum of forty-eight hours of recovery before undergoing the same training of the specified muscle group. Depending on several other components, the recovery time might be even longer than forty-eight hours. Typically, the maximum recovery time will be about seventy-two hours.

There are multiple approaches and considerations to recovery. The most popular and effective approach to recovery is active recovery, where athletes engage in an activity for a day or two with an intensity that is low.

Other major considerations in a person's recovery should be sleep, stress levels, nutrition, and hydration.

THE PURPOSE OF A WARM-UP BEFORE EXERCISE FOR ATHLETES

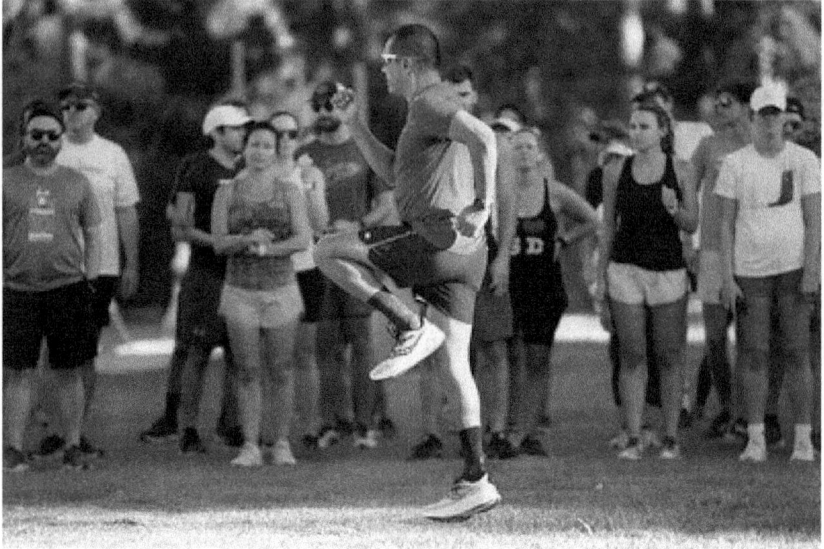

Running experts will always share with their constituents the primary purpose of a warm-up before running is to prepare an athlete physically and mentally for a training session or competition. At our San Diego Track Club workouts every Tuesday I prescribe runners to take part in a dynamic warm-up routine. A dynamic warm-up is defined as a sequential series of movements performed to physical activity, and I have found these exercises maximize one's own flexibility of the entire body.

After dynamic warm-up exercises are completed then static stretching is prescribed, and it is of little use if it's not done correctly. Stretching should always consist of warm-up exercises of a five to fifteen-minute period to allow muscles to gradually loosen and their core temperature to rise above 102 degrees. For example, an individual who experiences a tight muscle is susceptible to a muscle pull or strain. Athletes should perspire freely after their warm-up before they begin their workout. Wearing a warm-up suit will help accelerate the process of warming up and prevent athletes from cooling off again while they stretch. After the running workout, static stretching exercises is again prescribed to do.

Remember the reason you warm-up is to decrease the risk of injury and to enhance athletic performance and listed below emphasizes its purpose:

1. Raise the core body temperature to at least 102 degrees.
2. Rise in rate of metabolism.
3. Increase blood flow to muscles which translates to more oxygen.
4. Faster oxygen dissociation from hemoglobin.
5. Pre-overload of the muscles results in improved performance and working ability.

BENEFITS OF A PROPER WARM-UP

The sport of running is a unique blending of spiritual, physical, environmental, and mental challenges. It is both a sport and an experience, and one often overlooked ingredient that is vital to success in this demanding activity is a proper warm-up routine. A proper warm-up prepares you to fully use your physical, neurological, and psychological capabilities.

The muscular system must be properly prepared and so the temperature of the muscles must be elevated in order for them to work with optimal efficiency. The circulatory system must be properly stimulated in order for the most efficient transfer of oxygen and carbon dioxide. The working muscles must be saturated with as much oxygen-rich blood as possible prior to running. Furthermore, the body's cooling system must be elevated to its most efficient level. All of this cannot happen without a structured warm-up.

The neurological system must be prepared in order for the proper laying down of the technical neural patterns required for efficient running. With proper and consistent warm-up, the proper neural reflexes will be programmed. This will allow you to rely on properly conditioned reflexes for efficient movement. This also helps to allow for proper running rhythm.

The warm-up must also prepare you for the psychological demands of training and racing. You must have some sort of structured warm-up procedure that generally increases your focus until a total, relaxed concentration is reached. Without optimal preparation of the physical, mental, and neurological systems it's impossible to expect optimal performance in training or competition.

THE AMOUNT OF WARM-UP DEPENDS ON SEVERAL FACTORS

Albert Einstein's quote *"Persist Until Success Happens"* means having to keep on doing things until you achieve success, and this definitely pertains to warming up before running. Below are four factors that one must keep in mind when considering the amount of time devoted to warming up:

Individual Needs: Warming up is highly individual. Athletes who are less flexible or less skilled may need more warm-up to get ready. It's recommended you experiment and determine the right amount for you. Years ago, during my competitive track career while training for the 1,500 meters, a thorough warm-up was critical especially on interval days. A favorite workout of mine entailed running 400-meter repeats between fifty-eight to sixty seconds with one-minute rest. Now that I am approaching the age of sixty, my exercise regimen has changed and consists of a three-mile walk most days of the week so it's less intense than earlier in life when that same walk in the past would have served as a warm-up. One thing for sure is that your body will feel ready to go when it's thoroughly warmed up.

Intensity of Exercise: Maximal exercise which is going all out places great demands on muscle and joints and requires a thorough warm-up. Maximal exercise can take several forms. For example, sprinting 100 meters or serving a tennis ball is a type of maximal effort. Going for a two-mile stroll; however, is less severe and the walk itself can serve as a warm-up.

Environmental Conditions: You will need to warm up more in cold weather and less in warm weather. When it's cold out, warm up inside to avoid bundling up in clothing that you'll want to remove later.

Experience: When performing an unfamiliar activity, a more extensive warm-up can help prepare you for the unexpected.

WARMING UP IS GREAT FOR THE HEART

You probably know that warming up is important. It makes sense that the demands of exercise, especially intense competition, require the body's muscles and joints to be warm and limber. Athletes have long used warm-up to prepare their bodies for physical change.

Despite universal acceptance that warming up is good, what I find interesting, there is little scientific proof that it in fact improves performance or reduces injuries. This is because the need to warm up is ingrained in us, which makes it difficult for researchers to collect unbiased data. For example, try sprinting full speed on a cool day without warming up and your mind says to slow down.

However, one benefit of warming up has been documented. Research shows that warming up can decrease stress on your heart. If you try a very strenuous task like sprinting uphill without a warm-up, your heart muscle will probably not get enough blood flow and oxygen. Warming up will lower your blood pressure and increase blood flow to the heart. This could reduce the risk of a heart attack.

VARIOUS WARM-UP TECHNIQUES

During my coaching career I have been asked often: what is the best way to warm up? Many approaches have been used that include the following:

In passive warm-up, heat is applied to the body, such as in a sauna or with a heating pad or hot water bottle. Passive warm-up does little because deep muscles, which do much of the work during exercise, are unlikely to get warm. Furthermore, heating the skin can divert blood to the surface and away from deep muscles.

In active, general warm-up, total body exercise like brisk walking or jogging in place raises body temperature. Active warm-up is better than passive, but using a general approach may not warm specific muscles and joints.

With an active task specific warm-up, the skill employed during exercise or competition is used as a warm-up. A relief pitcher throws dozens of increasingly hard pitches in the bullpen. A swimmer does several leisurely laps, while football players may do short sprints at half speed. A runner might warm up by running for several minutes at a slower pace than the rest of his/her run.

Many people believe that stretching is a good warm-up, but actually working cold muscles before a general warm-up may cause injury.

HOW TO WARM-UP YOUR WORKOUT

No set schedule for warming up can be applied across the board. As a rule, begin with an easy-paced active general warm-up. One good basic routine involves four stages:

1. Walking
2. Brisk Walking
3. Jogging
4. Light Running

Most people should spend a minute or two in each stage, but if you're older or not in great shape, it's better to spend more time in the walking stages.

No matter what warm-up you choose, gradually increase the intensity until you sweat lightly. This should take about five to ten minutes, but don't do too much and stay below your workout or competition level. You don't want to exhaust yourself or reduce stored energy that you will need later. Your warm-up is too hard if you breathe heavily.

Next, do light stretching. For a demanding workout or for a sport that stresses a particular area, do a task specific warm-up. Start slowly, gradually building up to performing levels.

You want to warm as close to exercising as possible to avoid cooling off. If you're an athlete, competition doesn't always permit a timely warm-up, but do what you can to preserve building up heat. Furthermore, get up and move at every opportunity.

WARM-DOWN BENEFITS

While warming up is universally accepted, cooling down is often ignored. This is unfortunate because the warm-down can be just as important as the warm-up. Benefits of a warm-down routine include removing byproducts that are created during vigorous exercise. For example, lactic acid is removed from the muscles more effectively during cool-down exercises than when resting. Movement promotes increased blood flow that carries these products from the muscles, and you will recover faster from higher intense workouts. Removing byproducts is especially important to athletes like runners or swimmers who compete in two events with little time between events. Removing byproducts may not be as important for the average exerciser.

Warming down is important to everyday exercisers because it helps lower levels of adrenaline produced during vigorous exercise. Adrenaline that stays in the bloodstream while you rest can stress your heart. Being inactive after vigorous exercise also can cause blood to pool, especially in the legs. This pooling can lower blood pressure suddenly, which could cause lightheadedness and possibly inadequate blood flow to the heart. Warm-down exercises help circulate blood back toward the heart, because muscles squeeze the veins and thus aid in blood flow.

THE PRACTICE OF A WARM-DOWN IS A REWARDING EXPERIENCE

Just as important as a structured and thorough warm-up is a proper warm-down. Your body's muscles are highly used during a workout or race. A good warm-down will help the tendons, joints, and muscles recover in a quicker and more efficient manner.

A good warm-down brings about a gradual lowering of the body temperature and heart rate through slow jogging. This also helps the muscles to gradually re-synthesize lactic acid and remove harmful waste products. Static stretching also helps to relax fatigued muscles and allow for removal of waster products.

Consumption of carbohydrates and electrolytes within thirty minutes of a workout will take advantage of your muscles' greater ability to replace lost glycogen during this time. The replacement of fluids and the carbohydrate energy sources lost during the workout should be included in the daily warm-down in order to take advantage of this thirty-minute period of increased absorption. This quicker replacement of lost fuel will allow for a much fuller recovery.

Ingestion of vitamins C and E has been found to help decrease exercise-related muscle damage and speed up recovery. Remember, a better recovery will allow you to run at higher levels without experiencing the gradual onset of fatigue that many runners experience. By ensuring that you warm down you can guarantee that your running will be a rewarding experience.

HOW TO WARM DOWN?

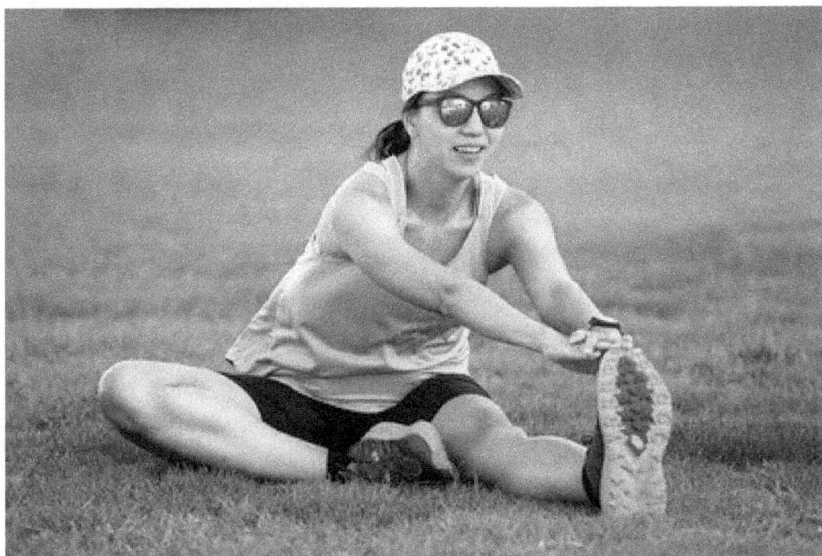

Cooling down generally consists of mild exercise similar to the activity just performed. After you have run several miles, an effective cool-down would be light jogging followed by a brisk walk. Continue until your breathing returns to normal and your pulse approaches its pre-exercise level. What worked for me tremendously in the past was spinning lightly on a stationary bike after a longer running workout.

Stretching is also an important component of the cool-down. After an activity that involves running, leg and low back muscles tend to tighten. Ignoring this tightness makes things worse, especially if you go right from exercising to the car or couch. Muscles may tighten further, causing stiffness and pain, so stretching after exercise helps improve flexibility because warm muscles tend to stretch more than usual.

During cold weather, do cool-down stretches indoors to slow the loss of body heat and help prevent a chill. It's also more comfortable to stretch in a warm environment.

GENERAL GUIDELINES FOR STRETCHING

There are seven guidelines for stretching that I prescribe and recommend you should always follow:

1. Always warm up before stretching. Five to ten minutes of biking, brisk walking, or mild calisthenics should do it.

2. Never stretch in a painful range of motion. Progress the stretch to a mild point of tension and hold that position as you relax into the stretch.

3. Do not bounce. For improvement in flexibility hold each stretch for twenty to thirty seconds.

4. Do not forget to breathe. Exhale as you relax into a stretch or just take shallow breaths. Do not hold your breath.

5. The stretch should be felt in the middle of the muscle. Avoid overstretching or forcing a stretch which could cause pain in or around a joint.

6. Stretching should be done on a daily basis after warming up and after any physical activity.

7. Be patient. Flexibility improves over a period of time when stretches are done on a regular basis. Do not expect immediate results.

ADDITIONAL FACTS ABOUT FLEXIBILITY AND STRETCHING

When stretching, make sure you feel the tension in the muscle you are stretching, which isn't necessarily the site of the injury. It's always recommended to not bounce and simply hold the stretch until you feel the muscles relax, and spend between twenty and thirty seconds stretching. It's best to stretch warm muscles, but it's okay to stretch gently when you haven't warmed up. Where stretching is indicated as part of the treatment for an injury, it's a good idea to stretch several times a day. Below are a few more facts about flexibility and stretching.

1. Technique matters in that there are three basic approaches to stretching used commonly. Ballistic stretching involves the momentum generated by the moving body part to produce the stretch. The second type of stretching is static stretching which involves gradually stretching through a muscle's full range of movement until resistance is felt. The stretch is held for a predetermined time and then the muscle being stretched is relaxed, followed by stretching that muscle even further. The final common stretching is contract-relaxing technique that involves performing an isometric contraction of the muscle to be stretched, followed by slow, static stretching of that same muscle.

2. You should not stretch to the point of pain. Flexibility cannot be developed while the stretched muscle is in pain, and besides you may get injured.

3. Generally speaking, women tend to be significantly more flexible statistically than men at all ages. These differences can be overcome by engaging in a properly designed stretching program for an extended period of time.

4. As you age, your level of flexibility tends to decrease, although such a decrease can be attributed more to a decrease of your level of activity rather than to the aging process itself.

5. It's important to not be discouraged with your stretching efforts because you are not progressing as quickly as you would like or are not as flexible as others. Remember, that flexibility is an individual matter, one that varies from person to person. Stay consistent and your efforts will pay off in the end.

SUMMARY OF IMPORTANT TIPS ABOUT FLEXIBILITY AND STRETCHING

We all should be aware now how flexibility is critical for the prevention of running injuries and athletic performance. Below is the summary of five important tips that are most beneficial for everyone to follow:

1. Achieving and maintaining an adequate range of motion in your musculoskeletal joints is important in reducing your potential for injury. An insufficient level of low flexibility in your hamstrings and lower back muscles is a major factor in the incidence of lower back pain.

2. The best time to stretch is just after a brief warm-up or dynamic exercises. Following such a schedule will increase your level of blood flow and raise the temperature level in your muscles, both of which are vital for muscle elasticity. Stretching cold muscles may tear them so you should always stretch after warming up.

3. One of the keys to maximizing your efforts to increase the level of flexibility is to perform two to three repetitions of each stretching exercise to the point of mild discomfort, holding each stretch for twenty to thirty seconds.

4. Begin your stretching routine by stretching the major muscle groups of your body first. Then, stretch the specific muscles involved in the activity in which you plan to engage.

    The sport of running emphasizes the quadriceps, hamstrings, and calf muscles of the lower extremities.

5. Make sure you isolate the muscles you want to stretch. If other parts of your body move while you are exercising, your stretching efforts

will be compromised and your risk of suffering an injury will increase.

With flexibility and stretching, stay consistent and your efforts will pay large dividends.

KNOW YOURSELF BEFORE SELECTING A RUNNING SHOE

It is important to realize that it is your feet that do the running and not the shoes. No matter how good a shoe is, if it doesn't fit with your feet and running style it will not work. In order to make a good choice you must first have some information about yourself. Below are three strategies and questions to ask yourself before choosing a running shoe.

EXAMINE YOUR FEET
- Are they wide or narrow?
- Do you have high or low arches?
- Do you have any problems like blisters, blackened toenails, or bent toes?

ANALYZE YOUR RUNNING FORM AND HOW YOUR FEET COME IN CONTACT WITH THE GROUND
- Heel first vs. toe first.
- Toe out vs. toe in.
- Inside vs. outside roll.
- Do you run level or up and down?

EXAMINE YOUR OLD RUNNING SHOES
- How do the outer soles wear?
- Did the midsoles compress unevenly?
- What is the shape of the uppers?

STEPS IN CHOOSING THE RIGHT SHOE FOR YOU

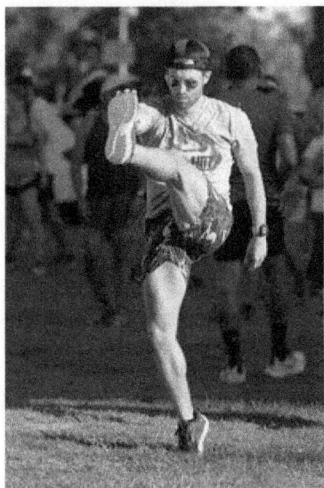

Another important step in choosing the right shoe is to gather information on what shoes are available. You can read the advertisements or talk to salespeople, but be skeptical since some might be motivated by sales rather than what is best for you. It's important to realize that a popular brand or a high price is no guarantee of a proper shoe for you. Below are a few more suggestions to follow:

LOOK AT THE VARIOUS KINDS OF AVAILABLE SHOES
- Find out what features are useful to your running style.
- Talk to other runners about what works.
- Observe what happens to various types of shoes.

TRY ON SEVERAL SHOES
- Comfort is the most important feature.
- Try them the way you plan to use them and with or without socks, orthotics, and insoles.
- Make sure they fit well so make sure ½ inch of space from end of shoe to end of toe when you stand in them. Furthermore, ensure you have a close fit from ball of foot to heel but room for the toes to move.
- Don't expect them to break in.
- Run in them to make sure they perform as you expect them to.

THREE DIFFERENT SHOE CATEGORIES

Due to the fact there are different shapes of feet and different amounts of foot motion, all of the shoe companies develop shoes that do different things. High arched feet are curved, and flat feet are straight. There are some shoes that are curved to meet the needs of high arched feet, and some are straight for flat feet. The rest of the shoes are made semi-curved, so it's recommended you select shoes for the shape of foot you fit and the kind of foot motion that is designed to do. Below are the three shoe categories for you to be aware of moving forward:

1. **Cushioned shoes** are made for feet which have no excessive motion, and they don't roll inwards or roll outwards. You will find they are not very shock-absorbing so instead they send shock up through the joints to the spine. Cushioned shoes are designed to reduce the shock.

2. **Motion Control** shoes are made for feet which roll inwards too much, they over pronate. Motion control shoes keep the foot lined up so the shoe can absorb the shock without breaking down too quickly.

3. **Stability shoes** are a compromise between motion control shoes and cushioned shoes. They inhibit extra motion but also supply a good amount of cushioning. They may have cushioned characteristics or stability characteristics.

RUNNING SHOE MYTHS

One of the many great things about running is its simplicity. You don't need a lot of equipment to run. Sure, retail supplies us the opportunity to purchase a slew of fancy running gadgets, but in the end, the only necessary piece of gear you need are a pair of running shoes.

How hard can it be to buy a good pair of running shoes? Like anything, advancement in technology and overzealous advertising can add unnecessary complexity and lead to shoe buying confusion and misconceptions.

TO HELP GUIDE YOU IN THE RIGHT DIRECTION, BELOW ARE 11 COMMON MYTHS ABOUT RUNNING SHOES, DEBUNKED.

- **Running shoes improve the performance of the foot.**
  False. Running shoes can enhance the performance of your foot, but you need to maintain good foot health via stretches and exercises to improve the performance of your foot.

- **A softer shoe offers better protection.**
  False. A softer shoe doesn't mean a better shoe. Sometimes a softer shoe can weaken tissue and cause overuse injuries. A good running shoe provides some cushion, but not too much.

- **New shoes are improvements on old shoes.**
  Definitely false. If you find a shoe that works for you, stick with it! Shoe companies are in the business of making money, so they will come out with new models often. However, shoe technology is already so advanced, and has been for years. So, find what you like and run with it!

- **The best shoe is the one that costs the most money.**

  False. The best shoe is the one that works best for your body type, your goals, and your wallet.

- **It works well for my friend so it will work well for me.**

  False. Running form is about as unique for each person as your fingerprint. Some people have a neutral stride, some roll outward (supination), some roll inward (pronation). Some people have long strides, some have short. In other words, pick out a shoe that is perfect for you and nobody else.

- **It fits poorly now, but it will "break in."**

  Yikes! If a shoe doesn't feel good when you try it on at a store, then don't buy it! A shoe should feel soft, smooth, and comfortably snug. Walk around the store for a bit. If you feel any rubbing, try on another shoe.

- **The salesperson knows what's best for me.**

  False. Trust yourself. Sure, a salesperson is likely a great source of running shoe knowledge and I recommend you ask questions and learn from them. However, nobody knows what's best for you except you.

- **The more gizmos a shoe has, the better it is.**

  False. First, don't believe everything you hear. A shoe can only do so much for you. The magic is in the engine that wears the shoe. So, choose wisely and don't be blinded by the latest and greatest advertisement schemes.

- **If I stick with a good brand, I cannot go wrong.**

  False. Just like cars, shoe brands make mistakes and come out with good and bad models. When you go to buy a running shoe, ignore the brand. Try on multiple shoes and go with what feels right.

- **The ratings in magazines are accurate.**

  False. Rating in magazines can be biased depending on the magazine, the author, and any supporting sponsors. Like anything, it is good to read through the ratings to gain knowledge, but don't put too much weight into the rankings when making a purchase.

- **Running shoes are the cause or solutions of injuries.**
  False. You are the cause and solution of injuries. You train too much or too little. You stretch too much or too little. You rest too much or too little. These are the causes of, and solutions to, injuries. Not shoes.

PREPARING YOURSELF FOR THE NEXT TIME YOU CHOOSE A SHOE

Once you have selected a shoe, you should allow yourself some time to get used to them. The fact that it's new will cause it to feel strange for a while. Give it some time before you assess your choice. By paying attention to how the shoe works for you will enable you to learn more about making a good choice the next time.

BELOW ARE A FEW TIPS TO FOLLOW:

- What happened to your shoes as you wore them?
- Where did they wear out the most?
- How well did they work with your feet and running form?
- Did they do what you wanted them to do?
- How could you improve on the choice you made?

"As we express our gratitude, we must never forget that the highest appreciation is not to utter words, but to live by them."

—John F. Kennedy

BREATHING TIPS

CAUSES OF SHORTNESS OF BREATH WHILE EXERCISING

Shortness of breath during exercise is not a matter of air supply as much as blood supply to muscles. When you exercise, the heart pumps more blood and the lungs take in more air to meet the muscles' increased oxygen demands and to remove the extra carbon dioxide given off by the working cells. During an unaccustomed sprint the heart and lungs temporarily cannot deliver oxygen to the muscles. While attending San Diego State University Kinesiology classes our professors taught us that muscles thus burn carbohydrates anaerobically (without oxygen) producing lactic acid, which can cause muscle pain and fatigue, experienced as a burning sensation. As your body neutralizes the lactic acid, more carbon dioxide is produced which makes you breathe faster to expel this gas. This results in feeling "short of breath."

One positive factor is as you become fitter through strenuous workouts you accumulate less lactic acid at a given level of exertion because you have raised your anaerobic threshold. Basically, you have enhanced the capacity of your heart and blood vessels to deliver oxygen to your muscles. Training effectively also enhances muscle fibers' ability to use oxygen so you can work more intensely.

Reference: https://www.pfizer.com/news/articles/science/lactic-acid-buildup-causes-muscle-fatigue-and-soreness

IS IT HAZARDOUS TO EXERCISE IN POLLUTED AIR?

The answer is yes. Since you take in more air when you exercise, you also take in more carbon monoxide and other pollutants. Thus, running when ozone levels are high may cause chest pain, coughing, throat irritation, and difficulty in breathing. The long-term adverse effects are unknown. If air pollution is a problem in your area — and for some reason, growing up in Solana Beach, California, there were times when air pollution was very high — I would exercise indoors or run early in the morning before pollution levels peak or in the evening after rush hour when levels fall again. It's important try to avoid running near heavy or even moderate traffic.

DOES GRUNTING HELP WHEN LIFTING WEIGHTS?

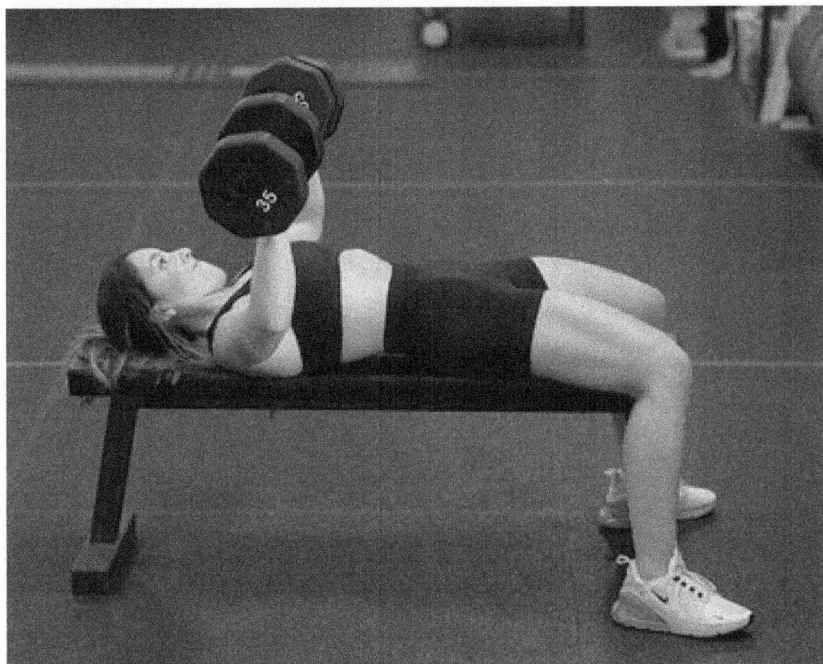

It may help, but it's dangerous. The grunts, along with other symptoms of pressure buildup such as bulging veins, come from forcing air out while your mouth and nose are closed. This process, called the Valsalva maneuver, can dramatically increase pressure in the chest area, cutting down on the amount of blood returning to the heart so drastically that dizziness, a blackout, or even a ruptured blood vessel can result. Don't hold your breath when lifting. A general rule to follow is to breathe out as you strain.

IS IT DANGEROUS TO RUN IN SUBFREEZING AIR?

If you're prone to exercise-induced asthma, cold air can bring on an attack. A light scarf or ski mask pulled loosely in front of your mouth can help warm up air. Another danger is dehydration, which will hinder the body's ability to regulate its temperature. When you're active, you lose fluids by sweating and particularly in winter by breathing. The dry winter air has to be warmed and moistened by the respiratory system. As you exhale you lose water; when you see your breath, you're seeing water droplets. Moreover, urine production is stimulated by the cold. Always make sure you drink water when running in these temperatures. Running under these very difficult conditions reminds us of the quote: "You have to fight through the bad days in order to earn the best days."

DOES INHALING OXYGEN FROM CANISTERS IMPROVE PERFORMANCE DURING STRENUOUS EXERCISE?

No! You may see some athletes inhale oxygen-rich gas at breaks in games or meets, but the practice has little or no effect on their performance. The hemoglobin in the red blood cells that transport oxygen to the muscles is normally 95 to 98 percent oxygen-saturated at sea level. Any small benefit from inhaling bottled oxygen would disappear after a minute or two of breathing normal air.

CAN I PERFORM BETTER BY BREATHING MORE EFFICIENTLY?

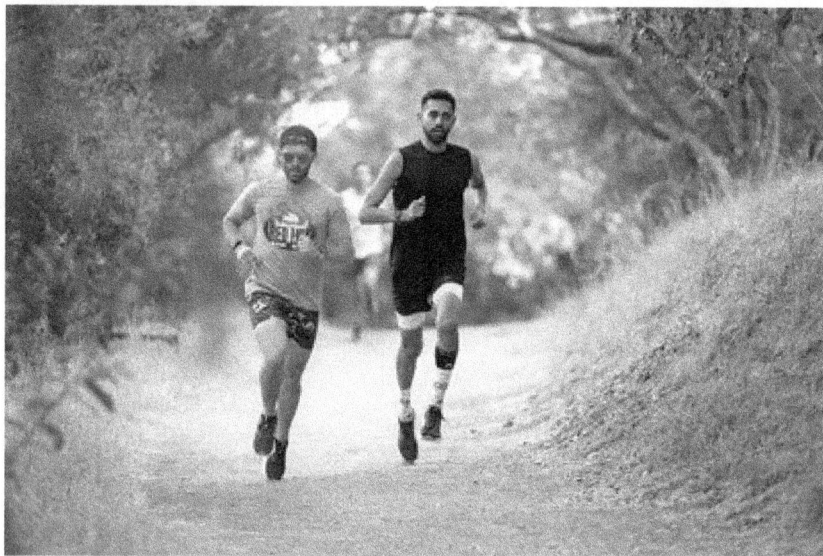

Improving your breathing while exercising takes time, but it comes automatically with training and improved fitness. If you don't run regularly, your breathing is probably quick and shallow when you work out. The more you train, the more efficient your breathing becomes — you breathe more deeply and find a rhythm that suits your activity. It's recommended the best approach to improving your breathing is simply not to think too much about it before you'll settle into an easy respiratory pace that suits you. Try not making too conscious an effort, which can throw off your natural breathing rhythm.

NOSE BREATHING WHEN RUNNING — A GOOD OR BAD THING?

There are many benefits to breathing from your nose since our noses are nature's natural filtration system. Nose breathing filters out dust and other allergens. Deliberate nose breathing also forces you to stay calm and thoughtfully breathe in and out, which is why it is commonly recommended for activities such as yoga, meditation, and deep breathing exercises. But should you exclusively breathe out of your nose during strenuous activity such as running? Absolutely not.

For those of you who have tried to only breathe from your nose while running, I'm sure you felt lighthearted in only a few paces. This is because when your heart beats fast, it needs oxygen. Oxygen is fuel. If your body isn't getting enough oxygen, it will start to shut down, causing dizziness, vomiting, vertigo, etc. When you do intense exercise, your body knows what to do and you automatically breathe out of both your nose and mouth. Don't fight your body's natural ability to efficiently inhale and exhale oxygen to fuel your strenuous running activity. Just breathe!

In summary, only breathing from your nose is good for slow, methodical activities and bad for strenuous activities such as running.

WHAT IS A "SECOND WIND"?

No matter how fit a person is, a few minutes into a bout of vigorous exercise you'll feel somewhat out of breath, and your muscles may hurt. I often share with fellow fitness enthusiasts in these instances your body is not able to transport oxygen quickly enough to the working muscles. Subsequently, the muscles burn carbohydrates anaerobically, which increases the output of lactic acid. You will find gradually, there is a change, and the muscles start to burn fuel (carbohydrates and fat) aerobically. You seem to be back in stride, and this is what's known as a second wind. The more one trains, the sooner you get your breath back and reach an aerobic steady state that you can maintain. From my personal perspective there is a feeling of pride and joy when your fitness improves in this regard.

WHY IS IT HARDER TO BREATHE AT HIGH ALTITUDES?

At San Diego State while competing in the sport of Cross Country we would as a team travel to Provo, Utah to race at our Conference Championships every year, so I discovered firsthand that when one runs up in the mountains and the altitude gets higher our breathing becomes more difficult. It's a fact that air pressure decreases the higher you rise above sea level. This means that the density of oxygen molecules falls with the pressure. This results in a lower concentration of oxygen in the blood which alerts the brain to increase your breathing rate. This faster rate is what you experience as difficulty in breathing. Endurance suffers because less oxygen is delivered to the muscles.

If you plan to exercise above 6,000 feet, approach it gradually. Planning at least one night's layover at a lower altitude is a good idea. In any case, do not attempt strenuous activity on your first day in the mountains. It's recommended you drink water to prevent the dehydration that accompanies rapid breathing of dry air at high altitudes.

FACTS REGARDING EXERCISE-INDUCED ASTHMA AND TREATMENTS

Three-time Olympic Gold Medalist Jackie Joyner-Kersee, who herself has asthma, once said, "*There are few restrictions on your life with asthma, as long as you take care of yourself.*" Exercise-induced asthma is an acute narrowing of the airway and contraction of the muscles surrounding the air passages that is started by exercise. Classic symptoms include chest tightness, coughing, wheezing, excess production of mucous, sore throat, and shortness of breath during or after exercise. The condition is much more prevalent than you might think. It's estimated that 12 to 15 percent of people in the United States have exercise-induced asthma. Furthermore, the condition is found in recreational and elite athletes. The symptoms are more likely and more severe during efforts that are intense or prolonged. For these reasons those who suffer from exercise-induced asthma should adjust their levels of intensity and duration accordingly. Cold, dry air causes more symptoms. An effective tactic is for individuals to cover their nose and mouth when exercising outdoors in cold weather. Anyone who suffers from exercise-induced asthma should seek the advice of a doctor who may prescribe medication as a preventative measure.

Before a run or race you need to warm up for about ten minutes. It's recommended you then start running hard which may cause the asthmatic response, triggering the release of adrenaline which then dilates the bronchial tubes. Run hard for five minutes then slow for five minutes and repeat this several times. Stretch and walk a little more and do this routine fifteen or thirty minutes before you race or run. It's important to remember the intensity of this warm-up results in a refractory period of about sixty to ninety minutes during which you should be able to exercise without an asthma attack.

Since cold, dry air can trigger asthma attacks, it's recommended you wear a surgical mask which you can purchase at a pharmacy or drug store. If you have allergies and notice more frequent asthma attacks during the spring and late summer, wearing a mask may help then too. Always be sure to inhale through the nose and be aware of air pollution and breathing at high altitude. Anxiety can worsen an asthma attack. Some experts recommend thirty minutes' relaxation or meditation sessions several times a week to teach you to relax during times of stress. If you cannot run for long without an attack, try running at intervals of three to five minutes with two to three minutes' rest between each interval. Eventually you should build up some endurance and be able to run longer. Exercise is excellent for asthma, but please be sure to consult a sports-oriented doctor about taking one of several safe, effective asthma medications that are now available to consumers.

"It's not what you do once in a while. It's what you do day in and day out that makes the difference."

— Jenny Craig

NUTRITION TIPS

ANTIOXIDANTS ARE GOOD FOR A HEALTHY, STRONG HEART

Health-wise, ultra-endurance events can sometimes lead to unhealthy behavior. While someone may look super fit on the outside, they could be damaging their heart and arteries on the inside. Research suggests that extreme exercise such as ultramarathons and Ironman distance triathlons are linked to lipid oxidation in the circulatory system. This oxidation can cause damage to cells, increased blood pressure, blood clotting, plaque formation in artery walls, and blood vessel constriction. This type of damage is also found after heart attacks, strokes, surgery, and similar trauma.

Recent research has found that taking antioxidant vitamin C and vitamin E supplements can prevent increased lipid oxidation. A study involving eleven of twenty-two runners preparing for a 50K ultramarathon were given daily supplements of 1,000 milligrams of vitamin C and 400 units of vitamin E for six weeks preceding their event. After the race, the runners who took the supplements only had increased lipid levels for a day, whereas those that did not take the supplements had increased lipid levels for a week.

This research enforces the fact that marathon runners should be taking supplements of vitamin E and vitamin C, if necessary. Vitamin C is easy to get from food or a small vitamin. Vitamin E, however, is a little more difficult since getting enough vitamin E from food along is challenging, which is why I recommend a vitamin E supplement.

The best food source for vitamin E are vegetable oils such as sunflower, canola, and olive oil. Nuts, sunflower seeds, and wheat germ are also good sources.

NUTRITIONAL NEEDS CHANGE WITH AGE

Unfortunately, the functions of the digestive system do not improve with age. Nutrient absorption tends to decline with age. However, older adults need fewer calories than they did in early adulthood and even with exercise older people experience some loss of muscle tissue and some reduction in metabolic rate. The challenge for older adults is to take in more nutrients with fewer calories. I realize as the years have passed by my own activity level has definitely slowed down. Nutrient needs that change over time include the following:

Sodium needs actually decline over time, as does the need for chloride. Older adults are more likely to experience high blood pressure with mineral imbalance.

Calcium requirements increase from 1,000 to 1,200 milligrams at age fifty since absorption declines and loss of bone mineral accelerates, especially for women. Calcium should be consumed throughout the day, rather than taking one supplement once a day. Too much calcium can contribute to kidney stones and other health problems. One serving of dairy or calcium-fortified foods gives you roughly 300 milligrams, and most people get at least 300 milligrams from the rest of their diet.

Absorption of vitamin B12 from food decreases in up to one third of older adults with a decrease in stomach acidity. B12 from supplements and fortified foods is more readily absorbed.

Vitamin D is an important hormone that keeps people healthy in many ways, including maintenance of strong bones. While people can make vitamin D given enough sun exposure, the body becomes less efficient at doing this with age. Add sunscreen, cold weather and D production drops. Cow's milk and soy beverages are fortified with vitamin D as are some breakfast cereals, types of orange juice, and yogurt. Adults seventy and over should consume 1,000 IUs of vitamin D per day. Meals and snacks that consist primarily of things your ancestors would recognize as food provide the best nutrition: fruits, vegetables, whole grains, and lean protein sources. Strive for five to nine servings of fruits and vegetables each day. Plant foods provide many helpful vitamins, minerals, and fiber. The minerals in vegetables help to promote a more healthful acid/base balance in the body which prevents calcium being drawn from the bones. A multivitamin and mineral supplement that provides the daily requirements for vitamins and minerals is good insurance so choose one low in iron unless you have been told by your healthcare provider to increase your iron intake.

A BREAKFAST MEAL FOR CHAMPIONS

There is no question that the most important meal of the day is breakfast, so below is a simple meal plan that will provide important nutrients with respect to improving your own athletic endeavors. One quick and easy breakfast of champions I personally enjoy is eating cereal with low-fat milk and adding a banana to it while drinking orange juice. Below are other types of foods you want to eat:

Carbohydrates: The best source of muscle fuel and carbohydrates should supply at least 60 percent of the calories in your diet. As already mentioned, a breakfast of cereal, low-fat milk, banana, and juice provides about 90 percent carbohydrates.

Iron: A mineral important for carrying oxygen from the lungs to your working muscles. An iron-rich diet reduces your risk of becoming anemic and experiencing needless fatigue during exercise. By drinking a glass of orange juice along with iron-enriched cereals, you will absorb more iron. All natural cereals such as granola, shredded wheat, or grape nuts have no additives, therefore no iron added to them. Combine them with enriched brands to enhance your iron intake.

Calcium: Derived from the milk or yogurt that you eat along with cereal. Calcium is important for strong bones and muscular contractions. Try to choose low-fat milk and yogurt as it's a heart healthier source of calcium than whole milk products.

Potassium: A nutrient that you lose in sweat. Bananas, orange juice, and whole grain cereals are potassium-rich foods.

Fiber: This indigestible portion of plant foods helps move foods through the digestive system, delays absorption of cholesterol and other nutrients, and softens stools by absorbing water. If constipation is an issue, fiber promotes regular bowel movements and thereby reduces the risk of unwanted bathroom stops during exercise. It's recommended you select raisin bran, bran flakes, all bran, corn bran, or any other bran cereals.

Breakfast can be a high carbohydrate energy booster for athletes who need to fuel and or refuel their muscles. Without this morning meal you will likely run out of energy, perform less effectively, and reduce your intake of nutrients that contribute to top performance. It's recommended you try these carbohydrate-rich meals for a high energy day.

1. Cereal, banana, orange juice, low-fat milk.
2. Muffins or bagels with jam, yogurt, dried fruit (raisins, apricots, dates, figs)
3. Pancakes, French toast or waffles with syrup, juice and low-fat milk.
4. Pita with 1-2 slices low-fat cheese, fruit and/or juice.

WHAT IS BEST TO EAT AT BREAKFAST?

I must admit that during my competitive running years, I did not always do a great job of eating a good breakfast. However, in a pinch, any breakfast is better than no breakfast, but some choices are better than others for your sports diet. Most athletes eat more than enough protein at lunch and dinner.

Breakfast is a convenient time to increase the carbohydrate intake. High carbohydrate choices include cold or hot cereal, pancakes, waffles, French toast, English muffins, bagels, toast, banana bread, fruit, juice flavored yogurt or whatever high-carb foods might be readily available for a non-traditional breakfast like pasta, baked potato, crackers, and thick crust pizza.

THE BEST CARBOHYDRATE SOURCES

A high carbohydrate diet translates into high performance workouts and races. It's fitting what Charles Swindoll says that *"Life is 10 percent what happens to you and 90 percent how you react to it."* Below are some of the best carbohydrate sources along with the listed calories for you to consider adding to your overall eating habits:

Food	Calories
1. Fruit juice (1 cup)	120
2. Dried fruit (raisins)	160
3. Corn on the cob	120
4. Banana, 1 large	115
5. Baked potato	220
6. Rice (white), 1 cup	223
7. Cereal (Ready to eat flakes), 1 cup	110
8. Spaghetti, 1 cup	160
9. Corn grits, 1 cup	146
10. English muffin (1)	150
11. Rice cakes (5)	200
12. Pita bread, 1 packet	106
13. Popcorn, 4 cups	92
14. Bread sticks (4)	154
15. Pancakes, three 4-inch	260
16. Pretzels, 2 ounces	222
17. Bagel, (1)	160
18. Kidney beans, 1 cup	186
19. Bread, 2 slices	160
20. Kashi, 1 cup	177

THE BENEFITS OF FRUITS AND VEGETABLES

My youth's mainstay of food was definitely meat and potatoes, and now as an adult I have a greater appreciation of fruits and vegetables in my diet. The reasons to eat lots of fruits and vegetables are numerous and not only do plant foods help lower dietary fat and control body weight, but they can also help fight disease. At first, nutritionists touted fruits and vegetables because they are packed with vitamins and minerals. It's recommended to eat plenty of plant foods to ensure a diet rich in vitamins, minerals, fiber, and other substances that might fight cancer, like antioxidants. Taking a vitamin mineral supplement or other supplement cannot match the benefits gained from eating food.

Recent research offers plenty of information and support to the pro-plant food faction. For example, two studies found that fruits and vegetables can help reduce the risk of stroke. Other studies reveal that eating onions lowers the rate of stomach cancer. Furthermore, eating a lot of foods rich in the substance lycopene primarily found in tomatoes and tomato products lowers the risk of prostate cancer.

THE IMPORTANCE OF IRON

Over the years, many runners that I have coached have experienced lower levels of iron. If you have restricted your red meat intake, you may have simultaneously restricted your intake of iron, which is an important mineral in red blood cells. Due to the fact iron helps carry oxygen to exercising muscles, iron deficiency anemia can pose risks when it results in fatigue during exercise. In order to eliminate the possibility of anemia, it would be wise to have your blood tested for hemoglobin and total iron binding capacity. Regardless of whether you're currently anemic, you can invest in your dietary iron intake to maintain appropriate iron stores. Some meat suggestions include small portions of lean beef and the dark thigh and leg meat of skinless chicken and turkey.

Non-meat sources of iron include fortified breakfast cereals, dried beans and legumes, dried fruits, and food cooked in a cast iron skillet. Unfortunately, these nonmeat iron sources tend to be poorly absorbed, so including vitamin C rich food with each meal can enhance iron absorption.

IMPORTANCE OF CARBS FOR YOUR MUSCLES

If you're filling up with greasy fast-food meals, you may be leaving your muscles unfueled. Fatty foods inadequately replenish muscle glycogen stores, and this leads to muscle fatigue. A high-fat diet simply cannot support a rigorous training program. If you must eat on the run, foods that are higher in carbohydrate such as thick crust pizza, submarine rolls for sandwiches, or extra rice can easily resolve the problem. Furthermore, my recommendation is to take easy to carry carbohydrate-rich snacks such as raisins, pretzels, fig bars, and juice boxes that can supplement your meals. You should make them readily available as emergency food for those days when you truly have no time to stop for a meal. I particularly enjoy fig bars, and this provides a very good nutrient in this regard.

The snacks will not only fuel your muscles but also help you to keep a higher blood sugar level, thereby providing energy for mental work and physical exercise such as running. Additionally, by eating these snacks expediently post-exercise you'll enhance muscle glycogen, since that's when muscles are most receptive to replacing the depleted glycogen stores.

MAKING EATING A PRIORITY

The book written by Md Kaif entitled *"Discipline is the fuel of achievement"* addresses the importance of how discipline is important in our lives and isn't just about controlling reactions or getting up early, but it pertains to abstaining from food. If you often skip breakfast and/or lunch because you think you don't have time, you're more than likely to feel droopy shortly thereafter because you've eaten insufficient calories to maintain a normal blood sugar level. Your brain, which relies on blood sugar for fuel, will think less clearly and may tell you that you are overwhelmingly sleepy.

The solution is simple: Eat breakfast and lunch! Chances are, the real reason you skip meals is lack of priority rather than lack of time. Remember, that the few minutes needed to eat these meals can make you more productive and ultimately save, rather than waste, precious minutes. If time is a concern, some quick and easy choices to help sustain you are as follows:

1. A glass of milk (Low-fat milk is recommended) or Juice
2. A couple of slices of bread (Whole grain is recommended)
3. A small bag of granola
4. A banana and yogurt
5. An apple and cheese
6. Crackers and peanut butter

CALCIUM IS CRITICAL FOR HEALTHY BONES

Getting enough calcium and protein is very crucial for women, who are susceptible to osteoporosis. Though activities such as running and weight training help build stronger bones, if you suffer from amenorrhea, you can lose bone mass despite regular exercise. That's because women with amenorrhea have lower levels of estrogen, a hormone that plays a key role in building and maintaining bone calcium.

An estimated 25 percent of women runners statistically experience amenorrhea at some point. Some are helped only by estrogen-replacement therapy. In other cases, a simple dietary change works, especially if you've been skimping on calcium and protein. Research suggests that the calcium RDA of 800 milligrams for women over the age of twenty-four is insufficient, particularly for athletes with amenorrhea. Around 1,200 milligrams, the equivalent of four servings of milk, looks to be more appropriate. As for protein, women vegetarians should know that a low intake may put them at higher risk of amenorrhea.

Be sure to get regular servings of daily products, calcium-rich tofu and greens, and calcium-fortified orange juice. This is something I personally paid attention to during my own racing career that provided rewarding benefits. Furthermore, eat lean meat and/or high-quality protein combinations such as pinto beans and rice. Try to avoid fiber supplements because these bind calcium and other minerals in the intestinal tract, thus decreasing the absorption of essential nutrients.

WHY CARBO-LOAD & STRATEGY FOR CARBO-LOADING

One of the most frequently asked questions I receive as a running coach pertains to the strategy of carb loading. The amount of glycogen stored in your muscles is directly related to the amount of carbohydrates in your diet and how much you run. For muscles to fill up with glycogen they must be somewhat depleted of their glycogen stores. This occurs with rigorous training. Diets that daily contain 60 percent or more of calories from carbohydrates will allow for the greatest storage of glycogen in the muscles.

Research with endurance athletes have shown that carbo-loading can improve both power and speed. Athletes ate either a normal carbohydrate diet or a high carbohydrate diet for three days prior to a three-hour cross-country race. The athletes who had carbohydrate loaded covered more distance faster at the end of the race compared with the other athletes who had not carbohydrate loaded.
Interestingly the athletes who loaded with 6g/pound/day stored no more glycogen than those who loaded with 4g/pound/day. In other words, there is a point at which muscle cells cannot hold any more glycogen. Subsequently, loading with carbohydrates will help, but overdoing it will not give you a greater boost.

Your diet should be high in carbohydrates each day, but this is not carbohydrate loading. Carbo-loading is a plan followed during the week immediately before a competition to give you a competitive edge. Keep in mind this is not for every athlete, but it is effective only during endurance competitions lasting ninety minutes or more. The basic strategy for carbo-loading is to rest your muscles before the race and to eat lots of carbs. Both parts of the strategy are important. If you do not rest your muscles before the race, you will continue to use the glycogen in storage, and never deplete your glycogen tank. I have seen some success from my marathoners in this regard toward their overall performances.

RECOMMENDED SERVINGS FROM FOOD PYRAMID GUIDE

The food guide pyramid provides a guide for daily food choices and shows that plant foods are the foundation of a healthy diet. This is something I teach during my Nutrition lectures at San Diego City College. With respect to the five food groups, it's recommended you use fats, oils, and sweets sparingly, 2-3 servings of milk, yogurt and cheese; 3-5 servings of vegetables; 2-3 servings of meat, poultry, fish, dry beans, eggs and nuts; 2-4 servings of fruit and 6-11 servings of bread, cereal, rice and pasta. The food guide pyramid de-emphasizes animal foods since they tend to be high in saturated fat. The body simply does not require a large serving to get these nutrients found in these foods.

Fruits and vegetables are not all created equal, so the question arises for us which plants have the biggest nutritional effect:

RECOMMENDED FOODS FROM THE FRUIT GROUPS:
- Oranges
- Strawberries
- Kiwi
- Cantaloupe
- Peaches and nectarines
- Grapes

RECOMMENDED FOODS FROM THE VEGETABLE GROUP:
- Broccoli
- Spinach
- Peppers
- Sweet Potatoes
- Onions
- Tomatoes

EATING FREQUENTLY IS ALWAYS A HEALTHIER CHOICE

Eating frequently during the day is good for you. People who keep their weight steady are usually those who eat at least four times a day and who do not skip meals. This approach may improve your work performance too, as studies have shown that eating a snack or a few hundred calories in the afternoon improved memory and cognitive skills later in the day.

On the other hand, skipping meals can leave you feeling drained, unable to concentrate, and lackluster about your evening workout. Furthermore, missing meals earlier in the day often leads to overeating in the afternoon and evening. At that point, you will be more likely to select foods that are high in fat, sugar, and calories. I share with my San Diego City College health students it's recommended to try eating around five times a day with three meals and two snacks. If you happen to have a busy schedule you need to plan ahead and get in the habit of stowing snacks in your workout bag or bring healthy foods to work for midmorning and midafternoon snacking. Dried fruit, energy bars, canned vegetable juice, and small boxes of ready to eat breakfast cereal are all good choices that are high in carbohydrates, fiber, vitamins and minerals.

SNACK FOODS NEGATIVELY IMPACT RUNNING PERFORMANCE

There are some important nutrition basics to keep in mind. Foods high in carbohydrates include grain, beans, breads, cereals, pastas, potatoes, fruits, and vegetables. Even though sweets and snack foods like desserts, crackers, and chips may have carbohydrates in them they are usually also high in fat. Due to the fact fatty foods will take up room in your diet where carbohydrates could go and because fats are slowly digested, it's best to stay away from them, especially before a running competition.

Back in 1993 I learned this the hard way while competing in an 800-meter race at the University of California San Diego. An hour before I was to race against the 1984 Olympic 800-meter gold medalist Joaquim Cruz, I ate a double cheeseburger from McDonalds — and needless to say, I ran poorly.

HEALTH ISSUES OF EATING FATTY RED MEAT

It's recommended to stop eating fatty red meat since too much fatty meat not only clogs your arteries, but it may also take the place of carbohydrates and may also take the place of carbohydrates you could be eating, which can lower stamina. This is still one of my personal struggles today since I tend to eat too much red meat. Lean cuts of beef, pork, and lamb can be easily included in your diet. It's recommended two to three-ounce servings of lean meat a day for a total of five to six ounces.

Lean meats are excellent sources of not only protein but also iron and zinc, two minerals particularly important for runners. Keep potions small. Simply slice a small piece of lean steak in thin strips, then stir-fry with veggies and serve with lots of carbohydrates-rich rice or add a little extra lean hamburger to spaghetti sauce.

PLANT FOODS ARE GOOD FOR YOU

Plant foods like fruits and vegetables should be the foundation of your diet and the reason for this is not because animal foods are bad for you — it's because plant foods are so good for you. If you eat at least the minimum number of recommended servings per day, you will be on the road to better health now and for the rest of your life. It's a heart healthy food so you will experience a better quality of life too.

SALADS SHOULD BE HEALTHFUL

Ounce for ounce, salad can be low in calories yet loaded with nutrition. However, if you add on ingredients such as blue cheese, bacon bits, or creamy dressing that thin salad can serve up loads of extra calories and grams of fat. I often share with college students when eating salads with those added ingredients it's the same nutritional value as eating a double cheeseburger. It's just important to keep salads healthful.

BELOW ARE A FEW TIPS:

1. Start with dark leafy greens: Lettuce, spinach, and mustard leaves can give you plenty of folic acid, vitamins.

2. Add protein: Choose from lean items such as grilled chicken or salmon, hard boiled eggs, black beans and chickpeas. Avoid fried or crispy foods.

3. Add on fresh veggies: For less than twenty-five calories a serving, you can get vitamin C, potassium, folic acid fiber and a variety of antioxidants. Be sure to choose a rainbow of colors including bell peppers, shredded carrots, onions, mushrooms, radishes, broccoli, and cauliflower.

4. Stick to low-calorie or low-fat dressings, or try mixing one to two tablespoons of light extra virgin olive oil with vinegar and fresh lemon juice.

CALCIUM FACTS TO FOLLOW

As a runner you can be confident in your bone health. Study after study has shown that weight bearing activities such as running increases bone mineral density in the legs and spine. Add adequate calcium to your regimen, and you're going to increase your bone health so provided are some calcium fun facts below:

1. Low-fat dairy products are the best sources of calcium. Dark green vegetables are good too, as are sardines and tofu.

2. Getting your RDA for calcium should not be a problem provided you are taking in calcium-rich food at each meal.

3. Calcium in the form of supplements is inefficiently absorbed, but ask your doctor or nutritionist about this alternative if your dietary intake is not adequate.

4. Sodium hampers calcium uptake so keep salt intake down if you're intending to increase your calcium. The American Heart Association recommends no more than 2,300 milligrams a day.

WHAT IS A CARBOHYDRATE & HOW CARBOHYDRATES WORK?

There are two different types of carbohydrates in foods:

1. Simple, such as sucrose Fruit (fructose) and Milk (lactose) sugars.
2. Complex Carbohydrates known as starches in breads, potatoes, beans, pastas, and cereals.

When you eat either of these types of carbohydrates, your body breaks them down into glucose, the circulating form of simple carbohydrate in your bloodstream. This is what your body uses for energy. After you eat any type of carbohydrate, your body either uses the glucose as energy right away, stores it in your muscles and liver, or if you overeat calories then are stored as fat. If the glucose is stored in your muscles, it is first transformed into glycogen, the storage form of glucose. When needed as energy, glycogen is taken out of storage and changed back into glucose.

When you exercise, you use both stored carbohydrate and fat for energy. Oxygen is needed to burn fat for energy, but not carbohydrates. At the beginning of exercise, adequate oxygen is not available in your body's cells, so your first source of energy is the glucose in your blood and glycogen in your muscles. As exercise continues, oxygen enters your cells, and you begin to use stored fat for energy. The longer you exercise, the more fat you use.

During my competitive years after a long, intense workout by running fifteen miles, I would start to fatigue. At that point, I returned to using carbohydrates for energy and the warehouse of glycogen in my muscles was called on. The more glycogen you have stored, the longer you can last.

REQUIREMENTS FOR IDEAL POST-EXERCISE RECOVERY NUTRITION

Ideal recovery nutrition requires two main components; however, these should be included with proper training, sleep, and stress management:

1. Proper hydration is needed throughout the day. The greater the temperature and humidity, the more fluids are required. Furthermore, for athletes who exercise in hot and humid weather or who exercise for an hour or more per day, sports drinks are the best chance for hydration and to keep blood glucose levels stable. Drinking sports drinks will help to spare muscle glycogen, especially in endurance events. To evaluate proper hydration, I often recommend that athletes weigh themselves before and after workouts. Ideally, if the athlete consumed enough fluids during a workout or event, he or she will find they have the same body weight before and after the practice or competition. An athlete should consume at least eight to ten fluid ounces of water or a sports drink for every pound lost after a workout or competition. Another method of assessing dehydration is urine color. Urine that is pale yellow is an estimate that a person is properly hydrated. Dark yellow urine usually means a person is dehydrated, whereas urine color that is clear may indicate over-hydration.

2. Food consumption is equally as important as hydration. Oftentimes after a workout or competition, athletes do not want to consume a lot of food. Nonetheless, consuming foods up to two hours post-exercise results in the best restoration of muscle glycogen. Thus, for athletes who cannot consume food right away after an event, liquid foods may be better tolerated after a workout or competition. Examples would be sport drinks, sports gels and water, nutrition shakes, chocolate milk, or fruit smoothies.

THE VALUE OF RECOVERY NUTRITION

One cannot underestimate the value of recovery nutrition with respect to the thousands of runners who complete marathons around the world. Recovery nutrition has become a popular phrase in the sports world and it's a mainstay for most marathon training programs and as important as everyone makes it to be. Recovery nutrition is important to working out because it's an accurate resource in restoring glycogen in the body, allowing for optimum performance from day to day. For the reason recovery nutrition allows for proper restoration of muscle glycogen, a person should feel strong each time he or she begins a workout or competitive event.

Other factors do come into play that include adequate sleep; seven to eight hours of sleep is recommended every night along with stress levels and proper training. Eight to nine hours of sleep is what I averaged most nights during my own training and competitive years. Nonetheless, even when a person is not obtaining the proper amount of sleep, for example, good recovery nutrition will still be helpful to the person's performance.

THE BALANCE OF CARBOHYDRATES, PROTEIN AND FAT

If you eat too many carbohydrates, you may deprive your body of protein and fat. The best balance for a sports diet is 55 percent to 65 percent of the calories from carbohydrates, 10 to 15 percent from protein, and 20 to 30 percent from fat. This means that meals are based on carbohydrates, not made up exclusively of carbohydrates.

Your protein intake should be two small servings per day to build and protect muscles. A few examples of a serving would be two tablespoons of peanut butter, three ounces of chicken, or half a cup of beans. It's recommended you should also include three to four servings of calcium-rich foods such as yogurt or milk for building strong bones. Furthermore, having a little bit of fat will balance your diet, providing essential fatty acids to assist in the absorption of certain vitamins. Limit or eliminate your intake of trans fats, and saturated fats should make up less than 10 percent of your total calories.

RESTRICTIVE DIETS ARE UNHEALTHY FOR OLDER ADULTS

Scientists have yet to discover a true fountain of youth, but regular exercise and a healthy diet provide the best chance for staying as healthy as possible as we age. The reason for this is that some of the physical decline associated with the aging process is accelerated by a sedentary lifestyle and poor nutrition. These unhealthy lifestyle habits may contribute to chronic illnesses like heart disease and cancer.

It's true that restrictive diets cause a loss of bone and muscle tissue that is difficult for older runners to regain. Such loss can accelerate the onset of osteoporosis and a progression into the frailty associated with old age. Restrictive diets rarely lead to successful long-term weight control, since weight is regained mostly as fat once the diet is ended. To lose fat it's recommended you increase your activity level of running and reduce food intake by eating less foods like desserts.

Strength training will help prevent muscle and bone loss. Fat that is lost very slowly is more likely to stay off and results in health benefits. An increase in activity will also improve health, even without any apparent change in weight.

YOUR MOST IMPORTANT MEAL IS BREAKFAST

If breakfast is the meal that you usually skip, and this is something that I myself need to do better, then make a resolution to change that habit forever. Without breakfast you'll be tired and hungry all day and if you have time to eat at home, it's easy to eat healthfully. Most calories are low in fat but be sure to read the nutrition label. Stick to 1 percent fat or non-fat milk. Toast fresh bread, bagels or English muffins and try topping them off with a low-fat jam, jelly or spread. Go light on butter and high fat spreads and eat only one or two slices of hard cheeses such as Swiss or cheddar. A piece of fruit or fruit juice will round out the meal nicely.

If you are heading out the door, a bagel with a slice of cheese or an English muffin with peanut butter and jelly make easy meals to go. If you'd rather eat out, try some of the fast-food restaurants but choose healthy eating options. Many now offer cereal with low-fat milk, low-fat muffins and pancakes.

MID-MORNING EATING CHOICES

Making the best of new and healthy foods take some planning. It's recommended always to review your daily schedule and figure out when you are hungry and then make a food plan that will fit into your lifestyle. Mid-morning is one time in the day that is challenging to prepare something healthy to eat. Prepare yourself to avoid the mid-morning sweets and you cannot expect your body and mind to perform at their best if you don't fill up with high performance fuel. It's recommended you pack a sack full of high carbohydrate treats to avoid grabbing high-fat treats and make sure to eat a snack a few hours before you exercise. Furthermore, drink plenty of fluids throughout the day.

Be careful in using vending machines since all selections are not equal. You are in good shape if you can get pretzels, low-fat popcorn, raisins, fresh fruit, juice, peanuts, low-fat granola bars and yogurt. If all else fails, plan ahead and bring with you some snacks from home. For example, my favorite is a bagel with peanut butter, and it makes a great snack.

MIDDAY MEAL PLAN IS CRITICAL & ARE ENERGY BARS FOR AN AFTERNOON SNACK BENEFICIAL BEFORE EXERCISE?

There are no excuses for skipping lunch anymore. You can stop by many fast-food restaurants and buy a low-fat meal. Fried foods soak up oil like a sponge so stay away from French fries, fried chicken, fried burgers, taco shells, and anything else on the menu that is fried. Be careful in eating a lot of foods that are prepared with saturated fats and lard.

Remember pizza is a good food source and pizza is actually a great food for an active person like a runner. The crust is high in carbohydrates, the tomato sauce has no fat, and the cheese is made from part-skim milk mozzarella. It's the meat toppings that can negate the good stuff, so it's recommended you stick to all veggie pizzas and don't add extra cheese.

Good deli selections are sliced turkey or chicken sandwiches with mustard instead of mayo. Even a peanut butter and jelly sandwich rates high marks and can be packed in a snap. Keep plenty of fresh fruit on hand to drop into your lunch or snack pack.

An energy bar is a convenient but expensive calorie source. You can get the same energy from snacks such as yogurt, a banana and juice, a bagel or fig cookies. You need to find out which foods settle best in your stomach. The popularity of energy bars has highlighted the importance of eating before exercise. Fueling within an hour before you work out boosts stamina and endurance.

EXAMPLES OF POST-EXERCISE SNACKS

Once an athlete is able to eat, the meal should consist of approximately 60 percent carbohydrates, 20 percent protein, and 20 percent fat. The carbohydrate can be a combination of low, moderate and high glycemic index foods. Athletes need to realize the importance of eating adequate energy and that there are times when that energy intake should be primarily from carbohydrates. It also allows an athlete to spread food consumption more evenly throughout the day. Below are examples of post-exercise snacks that work for many of the runners I coach:

1. 800 to 1000 ml of a sports drink

2. 500 ml of 100 percent fruit juice

3. A large muffin with a banana

4. 1 granola bar with a fruit yogurt

5. 3 rice cakes with a large apple

6. Bowl of cereal with low-fat milk or yogurt

7. 2 pieces of pizza

Recovery nutrition combined with proper training, sleep and stress management can lead to optimal exercise performance. When recovery nutrition is accurately implemented athletes will see a big difference in their overall performance and energy throughout the day.

THE IMPORTANCE OF TAKING VITAMIN SUPPLEMENTS

I have learned firsthand that if you are active and have a good appetite, you can get a lot of vitamins in your diet. Unlike an inactive person who might eat 1000 to 1500 calories per day, an athlete may top 3000 calories. By choosing wholesome foods, then, you can double or triple your vitamin intake. For example, if you drink 12 ounces of orange juice, you'll get 200 percent of the recommended dietary allowance of vitamin C.

If you eat fewer than 1500 calories per day, one multivitamin and mineral pill might be good. If you do not eat meat, iron and zinc supplements can be helpful. Note that some fortified breakfast cereals and energy bars provide 100 percent of the RDA for many nutrients. You do need to eat well even if you take a supplement and without a doubt, fruits and vegetables are the best sources of important nutrients. The ones with the most vitamins are oranges and orange juice, cantaloupe, strawberries, kiwi, bananas, green and red peppers, broccoli, spinach, tomatoes, carrots, and sweet potatoes. Those powerhouse foods provide vitamins and may also guard against aging, cancer, heart disease and other diseases.

YOU CAN MAKE HEALTHY CHOICES WITH PROPER PLANNING

Many of my San Diego Track Club runners will share with me their concern about eating healthier. It's recommended athletes plan ahead and take control of your meal, especially with respect to restaurant dining. Choose a restaurant that you know offers nutritious choices. Avoid all you can eat buffets and restaurants that specialize in fried foods. Watch out for the hidden fats in restaurant cooking sauces, butter, oil, mayonnaise, creams, and rich cheeses. Don't hesitate to ask questions about how the food is prepared. High-fat ingredients can often be eliminated from your meal, so it's recommended that you request that sauces, salad dressings, and sour cream be served on the side so that you can control the amount you use.

There might be many days when you don't get home until long after the standard dinner time. Who feels like making dinner at that point? You probably would rather reach for the cereal box than go through the hassle of preparing a cooked meal. However, cereal is a good choice and combined with low-fat milk and fruit, it can make an excellent late-night supper. By balancing the meal with some fresh vegetables and a slice or two of cheese on the side, you have a simple meal that will easily fill you up.

Another easy meal is the pasta found in the refrigerated case at your supermarket, combined with a red sauce. Stay away from cheese sauces because they are very high in fat. You can cook up the pasta and heat the sauce in only a few minutes. Stop by the salad bar at the supermarket and pick up a salad and soup to round out your pasta meal or as a meal in itself. Even if you are always on the move, with just a little bit of planning, your next meal will always be a healthy one.

NEW DIETARY GUIDELINES

The federal government's dietary guidelines for Americans completing the food guide pyramid are clear. The original dietary guidelines, which were developed by the US Department of Agriculture in the early 1970s recommended a diet low in fats, sodium, and alcohol and emphasized foods high in carbohydrates and low in sugar. The goals of these recommendations were to prevent disease and meet the body's needs for vitamins, minerals, complex carbohydrates like those found in starchy foods like bread and dietary fiber. These same guidelines are still being taught today.

Dietary guidelines for American's today suggest a diet with plenty of grain products, vegetables, and fruits. Specifically, these include breads, cereals, pasta, rice, potatoes, corn, dried beans, and all types of fruits and vegetables. The guidelines endorse a vegetarian diet as an alternative healthful way of meeting the recommended dietary allowances.

"Understanding the fact that we are essentially water is the key to uncovering the mysteries of the universe."

– Masaru Emoto

HYDRATION TIPS

DEHYDRATION EFFECTS YOUR RACE PERFORMANCE

During different periods of the year when climate changes and it's hot and humid we need to be careful when we run that we don't get dehydrated, which is an excessive loss of bodily fluids. Symptoms include thirst, dizziness, weakness, and nausea. Serious dehydration can lead to cramps, chills, and disorientation. In the case of severe dehydration, it's recommended you stop running, get to a cool place, and drink plenty of fluids.

However, the point is not to become dehydrated in the first place and you know you're getting enough if you void large volumes of pale urine at least six times a day. To determine how much liquid to take during a run or race you need to know your sweat rate and that can vary between one and four quarts per hour.

It's recommended you weigh yourself naked before a timed training run and then again after the run. One pound of weight loss equals one pint of water loss, and it's suggested you calculate your sweat rate and use this to determine your fluid needs during a run or race. For example, if you lose two pounds during an hour run that is two pints or thirty-two ounces. Consequently, you need eight ounces of water or sports beverage every fifteen minutes, and with respect to racing performance just know as little as 2 percent dehydration will have a negative effect on your race performance.

EXERCISE AND HYDRATION BENEFITS FOR RUNNERS

As I approach the age of sixty, I have felt the rigors of regular physical activity, and this has impacted my physical decline in profound ways. It's critical as one grows older, there are important adjustments being made to live your best life. Both endurance exercise and strength training improve stamina, blood sugar regulation, resting blood pressure, and body composition. Strength training improves muscle size and strength, and while metabolic rate declines with age, exercise expends calories, which allows you to eat more food and get more nutrients from your diet.

After exercise, enzymes responsible for muscle repair gear up for building muscle. Athletes often consume a protein and carbohydrate snack, beverage or meal within an hour of physical activity to maximize the anabolic effects of exercise. It's important to drink fluids. Thirst becomes a less reliable indicator of hydration with age so try to consume at least 8-ten eight-ounce glasses of water or other fluids daily and be sure to consume more water with exercise.

WHAT SPORTS DRINKS ARE BEST TO BUY

With warm days comes the need to drink water and in particular sports drinks. Several new products have appeared on the market over the last few years, and now they are filling the shelves in supermarkets and even showing up at some soda machines.

The one question from many consumers is: "What sports drinks are best to buy?" This is determined by your personal preference, but it's recommended you select one that contains around fifty to eighty calories per eight-ounce serving. Any more and the carbohydrate concentration will inhibit fluid absorption. It's suggested you test different brands during training, particularly on long runs, and monitor what works best for you. You will find some are slightly carbonated, which is fine if that is your preference. Whatever you choose, a sports beverage can be a valuable part of your refueling and rehydrating routine, and I personally enjoy consuming Vitalyte.

DOES FORTIFIED WATER OFFER ANY ADVANTAGES OR BENEFITS?

Fortifies or enhanced water contains vitamins, but each bottle costs more than $5. For less than a dime, you can get pretty much the same thing by washing down a multi-vitamin/mineral supplement with a glass of water. Fortified water usually contains more sugar and more calories than might be expected and an eight-ounce serving of one popular water beverage.

If someone who drinks a twenty-ounce bottle gets 32.5 grams of sugar this becomes an issue for those who are trying to lose weight, these calories only add to their calorie budget. For years, as a coach I am approached by athletes who share their own frustration in losing weight even though they are jogging for over two hours at a time. Individuals who eat a balanced diet have no need to drink water that is fortified with vitamins so the best way to get vitamins and minerals is by eating fruits, vegetables, and other wholesome foods. Many water beverages offer an alluring array of other enhancements in the products live up to their advance advertisements. The best way to get fluids is to drink plain, old-fashioned water, a habit that I can personally do better on.

RECOVERY DRINKS BY DEFINITION

Recovery drinks are high carbohydrate drinks with significant amounts of protein, small amounts of fat, vitamins, minerals, and electrolytes. The calorie counts range from 200 to more than 300 per eight ounce serving. They come in a variety of flavors in either cans or mix-it-yourself powders.

Recovery beverages were developed after research showed that adding some protein to the carbohydrates athletes consume post exercise facilitated glycogen storage in muscles. The most widely available brands include products like Gatorade but there are many others. It's recommended you drink these products immediately following exercise recovery. I recommend you experiment with different beverages before deciding the right beverage for you.

DIFFERENCE BETWEEN WATER AND SPORTS DRINKS

For some people water may seem boring, but research by the makers of sports drinks has shown that active people tend to drink more fluid it if tastes good. Given the choice between a tasty sports drink and plain water the sports drink will disappear faster. A sports drink can, if you are an endurance athlete, mean better hydration not only because you drink more fluid, but also because your body absorbs sports drinks slightly faster than water. Furthermore, sports drinks replace carbohydrates that help fuel your muscles.

Many of my fellow running coaching colleagues believe that you only need the benefits of a sports drink during endurance exercise that lasts more than sixty to ninety minutes. I agree. A recreational runner who works out for less than an hour has no need for sports drinks. It's recommended you make sure to drink enough to stay hydrated for your health and your athletic performance.

FLUID INTAKE IS IMPORTANT IN PREVENTING DEHYDRATION

The rapid loss of body weight that can occur during a workout is not fat loss, it's fluid loss from sweating. Some will say it's dehydration. When you lose weight during exercise, you are losing fluids that your body needs in order to function properly. The best step to take is to drink enough during your workout to minimize that weight loss. A smart hydration plan takes into consideration your sweat loss and how much fluid you will need to drink in order to replace that sweat loss.

An easy way to determine this is to pay attention to the difference in body weight before and after exercise. It's recommended you weigh yourself before and after your workout, and if you weigh less drink more during future workouts with the goals of finishing exercise within 2 percent of your starting weight. For example, after your workout a 140-pound man should drink during exercise to keep his body weight between 137.5 and 140-lbs after his workout.

If you happen to weigh more then drink less during your next workout. From time to time, it might be a good idea to monitor your weight in this regard, and I have witnessed much success when my own athletes have executed this approach.

FLUID-REPLACEMENT DRINK FACTS

If you have no time for a pre-workout meal or cannot take in anything solid before your morning run, deciding which product to buy and when to use it can be so overwhelming that you could end up with empty hands. Below are facts about fluid replacement drinks.

Fluid replacement drinks are water, simple sugars, and a small number of electrolytes and flavorings. They are available in a variety of flavors, and most have fifty to one hundred calories and fourteen to twenty-five grams of carbohydrates per eight-ounce serving. Sports drinks are designed to maximize fluid absorption and supply energizing carbohydrates for performance enhancement. If you like their taste, you will likely drink more and stay better hydrated than you would on water. Products like Gatorade, PowerAde, and Cytomax are a few of the major brands but there are at least ten to fifteen others on the market.

Hydration is key to staying energized and there are minimal nutritional differences between most brands of sports drinks so it's critical to choose the one you find the tastiest. Whichever brand you choose it's recommended you drink four to eight ounces every fifteen to twenty minutes during exercise. It's best for most athletes and again especially those who exercise for more than an hour at a time.

ARE YOU TAKING ENOUGH WATER FOR YOUR HEALTH?

Because water is fundamental for survival, you need to drink enough water every day to replace the amount you lose through urine, sweat, and the air you breathe. Even if you don't exercise, it's estimated you lose about twelve ounces of water per day with simple breathing and another twenty-four ounces through the skin. Then add strenuous exercise and you could lose up to four pounds of water or two quarts per hour.

An even easier way to find out if you are getting enough water is to simply check your urine. If you urinate a significant amount regularly throughout the day and if your urine is clear colored, you are drinking enough. For some athletes this may mean drinking twelve to sixteen glasses of water and for others they may need to drink far less; however, urinating about every two to four hours is fine. If you have to visit the bathroom every half hour, you might be needlessly drinking more than required.

DEHYDRATION AND ITS NEGATIVE EFFECTS

A severe lack of water can play havoc with your body's ability to function at its best. During the first few hours of water deprivation, water is lost primarily from blood volume. The reason is about 90 percent of your blood should be water; one danger of getting dehydrated during exercise is it will take longer for nutrients to be transported to and from your muscles. Subsequently, your sports performance will suffer.

With continued water deficit, your cells lose water, resulting in cellular dehydration so when cells become overheated, they experience dramatic changes that can impair how they work. Water loss of 9 percent to 12 percent of your total body weight can be fatal. Be careful!

FACTS TO KNOW ABOUT WATER

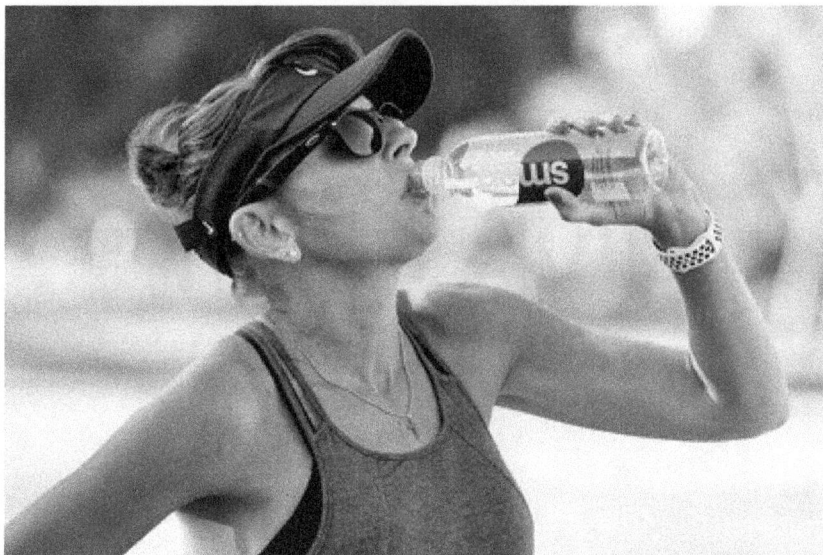

Water is a basic nutrient and is essential for you to live and for your body to function properly. You can survive for weeks without food but only for a few days without water. Water makes up about 60 percent to 70 percent of your body weight. Muscle tissue is 70 percent to 75 percent water and in comparison, fat has only about 10 percent to 15 percent water. Water has very important functions in your body so below are a few facts to keep in mind moving forward.

1. In saliva and stomach secretions it helps digest food.

2. In body's fluids it helps lubricate the joints and cushion organs and tissues.

3. In blood, it transports carbohydrates, facts, proteins, hormones that regulate metabolism and oxygen to the working muscles. It also

carries away waste products such as carbon dioxide, ammonia, and lactic acid.

4. In urine it carries waste products out of your body. Exercise increases the production of wastes and dark urine carries a lot of wastes.

5. In sweat it removes the body heat you generate during exercise. Water helps regulate body temperature by absorbing the heat from the muscles and transporting it to the skin's surface. Loss of a pound of sweat equals about 250 calories of heat lost.

ADDITIONAL INFORMATION REGARDING SPORTS DRINKS

Drinks like Gatorade and Exceed provide carbohydrates and salts in addition to water. Unless athletes are exercising over two hours, they need only water. Muscles contain enough glycogen to fuel a two-hour effort and after two hours the carbohydrates in sports drinks will replace the depleted energy stores.

As for salt, not enough is lost in sweat to require replacement in a concentrated form such as a salt pill. A normal diet should replace lost salts. It's critical athletes are drinking enough to get the water they need that includes five to eight ounces of a 4 to 10 percent solution sports drink every fifteen minutes. The sugary sports drinks do come in handy after exercise when replacing fluids and carbohydrates contributes to a fast, complete recovery from a workout. Immediately after a long workout, the body is most receptive to producing muscles' glycogen and glycogen supplies, the fuel to exercise again later. Furthermore, a balanced meal will replace vitamins, minerals, and salts. Sports drinks may be a way to ensure quick replacement if a proper meal is hours away.

IT'S IMPORTANT TO PAY CLOSE ATTENTION TO THIRST

Thirst is your body's way of telling you it wants or needs liquids. Under normal resting conditions, thirst does an adequate job of helping you keep water balance. If your body fluids become abnormally concentrated because you're lacking water, your brain receives a signal that makes you feel thirsty. This usually occurs after you are already a little dehydrated.

In some circumstances, you will find the thirst mechanism isn't reliable so it's possible among athletes thirst can be blunted by exercise and overridden by the mind. This is why extremely active athletes should drink more than required to satisfy their thirst. From personal past experiences I have seen firsthand where long-distance runners misjudged their water intake that led to dehydration and negative impact on performance and reminds us all of Brandon Mull's quote, "Smart people learn from their mistakes; however, the real sharp ones learn from the mistakes of others." It's in those moments when witnessing others falter that it works to check yourself periodically that you are taking in enough water. The thirst mechanism in young children and older adults may also lack the sensitivity needed to match their fluid needs so they may not feel thirsty even though their bodies need fluids.

IS IT BAD NOT TO DRINK EIGHT GLASSES OF WATER EVERY DAY?

With as many sports nutrition ideas it's no wonder people become confused. Sometimes the results from a new study on food can completely contradict what you may have previously heard, leaving you more confused than ever. One question often asked is regarding is it bad to not drink eight glasses of water every day. Keep in mind you don't have to drink water to fulfill your fluid requirement. Many foods are water-filled such as juice, oranges, lettuce, soup, yogurt, milk, and vegetables. Even coffee and tea supply water, but they tend to increase urination.

For reasons your fluid need is based on the calories you burn, you may need more than the proverbial eight glasses per day so it's recommended one ml of water per one calorie burned. For an inactive person who requires about 2,000 calories per day, this comes to 2000 ml or about eight glasses. Athletes who burn off 3000 to 6000 calories per day need even more fluids, so the easiest way to tell if you are drinking enough is to again check your urine and it should be clear in color.

TIPS TO PREVENT DEHYDRATION

To find out how much fluid you are losing, it's recommended you weigh yourself before and after exercise. Any weight loss in that short amount of time or over one or two days is water loss. Below are other tips to help prevent dehydration:

1. Be sure to drink plenty of water before, during, and after exercise.

2. Attempt to keep water cool because cool water leaves the stomach most quickly.

3. It's important to monitor your urine. Scant or unusually dark urine can indicate a fluid shortage in the body.

4. Do not rely on thirst, since thirst lags behind the body's need for water. It's recommended to make drinking water a habit and plan your long runs so you pass water fountains or a friend's house where you can stop and drink.

5. Schedule your long runs for the coolest time of day. The early morning or evenings when the sun is low is the best time.

Many athletes have asked how much water they should drink. The guideline used to be five ounces of water every fifteen minutes, but in hot weather that may not be enough. It's recommended runners drink as much as possible, but be careful and balance water with electrolytes. This is critically important, so you avoid the risk of hyponatremia, which is a lower than normal level of sodium in the bloodstream.

THE VALUE OF REPLACEMENT DRINKS

To avoid dehydration, particularly when exercising, you need to keep your fluid level. Pre-hydration consists of consuming fluids before exercise, especially before exercising in the heat it's a good idea. Drink more fluid than normal one to two days before an event to ensure full hydration. Approximately fifteen to thirty minutes before your running event, drink twelve to twenty ounces, letting comfort be your guide.

It's recommended to drink a commercial sport drink or salted water because water alone without sodium or other additives may stimulate urine production. Increased urine production not only undermines your efforts to avoid dehydration but can be inconvenient if not embarrassing during a competitive race. Back in 2007 during the Port Angeles marathon, I personally experienced this issue for the need to urinate often so proper planning in this regard is most beneficial.

WHAT TO DRINK DURING EXERCISE?

Guidelines for what to drink during exercise are less clear. The purpose of drinking during exercise is to provide water that can be used for sweat. The more readily water can be turned into sweat, the better, and water alone is generally the drink of choice because it moves most rapidly through the stomach and increased urine production is not likely to occur. When electrolytes and carbohydrates are added to water, it takes longer for water to be absorbed and used as sweat.

The benefits of drinking electrolyte and carbohydrate fluids during exercise must be weighed against the delay in absorption. Recent research suggests that low concentrations of additives delay absorption minimally, but more research is needed before firm guidelines can be set up. Furthermore, it appears from this same research that drinking electrolyte and carbohydrate fluids may not be necessary unless you exercise for one hour or more.

The best way to ensure a proper concentration of electrolytes as replacement fluids is to consume commercially available drinks that are approximately equal to the electrolyte content of sweat but with a glucose concentration of no more than 6 percent to 8 percent such as Gatorade or exceed fluid replacement and energy drink. The added carbohydrates in such drinks may help you retain the fluids and simply adding water is helpful.

EVERYTHING YOU NEED TO KNOW REGARDING FLUID-REPLACEMENT DRINKS

The science of hydration sure has changed since the days I competed in the early to mid-1980s at Saint Augustine High School and San Diego State University. Back then, my teammates only knew to drink water, so I recognize that deciding which fluid replacement drink to buy can be overwhelming. Here are a few suggestions on what fluid replacement drinks are and how to use them:

Fluid-replacement drinks are water, simple sugars, and a small amount of electrolytes and flavorings. They are available in a variety of flavors and most have fifty to 100 calories and fourteen to twenty-five grams of carbohydrates per eight-ounce serving.

Sport drinks are designed to maximize fluid absorption and supply energizing carbohydrates for performance enhancement. If you like its taste, you are likely to drink more and stay better hydrated than you would on water. As a result of hydration been the key to staying energized and there are minimal nutritional differences between most brands of sports drinks, choose the one you find the tastiest.

Whichever brand you choose, drink four to eight ounces every fifteen to twenty minutes during exercise. Fluid-replacement drinks are best for athletes but especially those who exercise more than an hour at a time.

WATER RECOMMENDATION FOR ATHLETES

The body's need for water is second in importance only to its need for oxygen. Water plays an essential role in the human energy system. The more we expend, the more we need. The following recommendations can help ensure your body has adequate water to keep you working in top condition:

1. Drink eight to ten eight-ounce glasses of water or other fluids daily.

2. Start drinking before you feel thirsty, since during activity the body loses water faster in sweat than it can absorb into the digestive system.

3. Use water to cool your skin during activity.

4. Wear light, loose clothing in hot weather to help sweat evaporate.

5. Weigh yourself before and after activity, replace the water you have lost with cool fluids.

6. Don't count on thirst as an accurate guide to your water needs. You will quench your thirst long before you replenish your body supply.

7. Don't try to lose weight by not replacing water lost during activity.

8. Don't wear rubberized clothing designed to increase sweating. It cannot help you lose weight as it just prevents sweat from evaporating.

KEEP YOUR BODY RUNNING SMOOTHLY BY DRINKING WATER

Running during hot summer months can leave you drained and low in energy and this includes during cold winter months one should stay hydrated. You definitely need to drink a lot of liquid during these times, but you may not realize just how vital it is to do it. Taking in too little fluid can be disastrous for your running and your health. Drink the right amount of the right beverages and you'll feel great and run fast. Drinking the adequate consumption of water is something that personally is a challenge. I don't necessarily associate dehydration and cold weather, so I am less likely to make a point to stay hydrated during the winter than during the summer.

BELOW IS HOW WATER WORKS TO KEEP YOUR BODY RUNNING SMOOTHLY.

On average, the human body is more than 50 percent water. Runners average around 60 percent. This equals about 120 soda cans worth of water in a 160-pound runner. A runner's watery physique results from physiological adaptations brought about by running. For one, running builds lean muscle tissue and reduces body fat; lean tissue contains more water than fat tissue does.

Another reason for your full of water state is one's own expanded blood volume. This occurs as you become physically fit and serves to improve oxygen and nutrient delivery to working muscles. The extra blood also helps remove wastes produced by muscles during exercise.

HELPFUL TIPS FOR WATER INTAKE

If you want to make sure you are getting enough liquids, increase your water intake. Below are some helpful tips:

1. If you are hot, cold water will better cool your body than room temperature water.

2. If your tap water tastes bad, try a water filter or bottled water for a consistently pleasant flavor.

3. Keep a filled water bottle by your side at work and take water breaks instead of coffee breaks.

4. Stock your refrigerator with a pitcher of tap water or possess bottles of spring or sparkling water. For added flavor, add lemon slices.

5. Carry a bottle of water to the gym so it will be ready for fluid breaks. To keep it cold and refreshing, wrap it in a towel or keep it in a small cooler.

6. If you work out in hot weather, especially if you bike, you can drink from a water bottle that has been stored in the freezer. Water will thaw in the heat at about the same rate you want to drink during exercise.

THE CAUSES OF DEHYDRATION

People who exercise in the heat must be careful to avoid dehydration and excessive water loss from the body. Extreme dehydration can result in heatstroke and even death if exercise is not stopped immediately and heat reduction measures started. Dehydration can be avoided easily by drinking plenty of fluids before, during, and after exercise.

Ideally, water lost as sweat should be replaced quickly but this does not always occur. Fortunately, your water reserves are substantial and can cover short-term deficits. Excessive water loss critically reduces your water supply, resulting in dehydration.

Dehydration can be acute, which means extreme water loss over a period of hours, or chronic, which is water loss that is never completely replaced, and the water debt grows over time.

The major consequences of dehydration are reduced blood volume. When blood volume is lowered, circulation is affected and the delivery of oxygen to the working muscles is reduced, resulting in fatigue. Lowered blood volume means that less blood is circulated through the skin. This hinders heat loss and further contributes to fatigue. When dehydration is extreme and too much blood volume is lost, your body stops sweating to preserve the remaining blood volume. Without the ability to sweat, your core temperature can go up, resulting in heatstroke.

A VALUABLE OPTION IS WATER

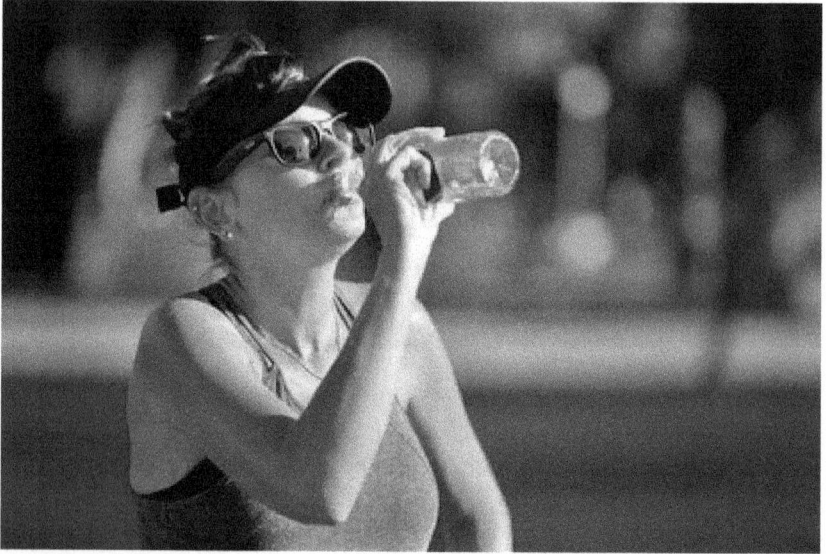

The beverage aisle in any grocery store overflows with drinks: bottled waters, bottled teas, juices, and many other selections. There is also plain tap water and so this begs the question, "What is best for you?" Tap water is fine and it's cheap. Furthermore, local municipal water supplies must follow strict safety regulations so if the water out of your faucet tastes okay than do it.

Many consumers choose bottled water, which generally tastes better than tap water because bottlers use ozone as a disinfectant instead of chorine. The general perception is that bottled water is better for you than tap water and safety regulations are higher for municipal water than bottled. Some bottled water may offer minerals such as calcium and magnesium, but if you live in an area that has hard water, your local water probably has more minerals than bottled water does.

Bottled teas and juices are tasty, thirst-quenching options but watch for caffeine, which can increase body water loss by increasing urine production. Furthermore, you may be taking in unwanted calories as many of these beverages have a high content of sugar or corn syrup.

DOES CAFFEINE IMPROVE RUNNING PERFORMANCE?

Caffeine is a stimulant to the central nervous system and is the most widely used drug in our society today. Caffeine is a component of tea, coffee, chocolate, and soft drinks, in addition to pills to lose weight and combat drossiness. It has no significant nutritional value.

Worldwide interest in the use of caffeine as a performance enhancer for running was historically inspired by two studies published in 1979. In these studies, caffeine produced significant improvements in cycling endurance. To this day there have been several studies conducted that have shown caffeine increases performance in cycling and running for durations of roughly five to twenty minutes. Drinking caffeine is a common practice among many of our elite endurance runners, and during my running career my ritual was to drink one cup of coffee before competition. At this time, it doesn't appear as if caffeine improves sprint performance.

Low doses of caffeine do not pose any serious risks for healthy individuals; however, when consumed in high doses, caffeine has the potential for many adverse side effects. Some of these symptoms include anxiety, tremors, inability to focus, diarrhea, insomnia, and headaches. Since caffeine is a diuretic there has been some concern that it can increase the risk of dehydration. This definitely presents problems during physical activity, especially in a hot, humid environment.

THE IMPORTANCE OF FLUID REPLACEMENT - DRINK UP!

It's understood sweating keeps you cool but losing all that fluid lessens the efficiency of the internal operations of your body. Most runners fall short on fluid replacement and only manage to replace about half their sweat losses. If you don't take in fluids as you sweat, your blood actually thickens. This makes your heart pump harder and slows oxygen and nutrient delivery to exercising muscles and as a result your body suffers.

As you dehydrate and your pace slows, you may become dizzy, weak, or nauseated. Eventually, in more severe conditions you may cramp up, get chills, or even hallucinate. Some of these symptoms may even occur at the office or at home as your fluid needs are not met and furthermore doesn't always conveniently show up on your run.

Your fluid needs depend on many factors, including body size, fitness level, training schedule, and dietary factors such as caffeine and alcohol consumption, both of which increase fluid loss from the body. The question of how much fluid you need is an individual matter, so it's recommended that you monitor urine color and frequency of urination. Pale yellow urine is a good sign that plenty of fluid is on board for waste excretion. Frequent urination is another good sign that you're getting enough fluid.

Spread out your fluid intake over the day to keep body water levels steady and to ward off the threat of dehydration. Remember to drink past the feeling of thirst, since that sensation shuts off quickly once you begin drinking. In fact, it actually turns off before you've replenished lost fluids.

BEING HYDRATED IS IMPORTANT BUT DRINKING TOO MUCH IS DANGEROUS

We have all heard the advice to drink plenty of water and we have been told to drink as much as you can. Don't wait until you are thirsty, by then it may be too late. However, the USA Track and Field Federation says that endurance athletes consuming huge amounts of water over the course of a long event may risk seizures, respiratory failure, and even death from drinking too much.

It's recommended that instead of drinking as much as you can, the existing guidelines say runners should drink when they are thirsty. People in long races may want to weigh themselves before and after long practice runs to see how much they lose from sweating, then drink that amount when they race and no more. The problem with the advice of water gorging is that the consumption of too much water dilutes their blood and their sodium levels plummeted a condition known as hyponatremia.

The problem occurs in any endurance event that gives people the time to drink. It appears among people who compete in marathons and Ironman Triathlons. Interestingly, hyponatremia is not a problem for elite marathon runners because they run too fast to drink too much. This problem increases with the slower runners so it's critical to be hydrated but not drink too much. No one has ever died of dehydration when running a longer endurance event, including marathons, but there are always a few runners every year that die from hyponatremia. Be careful!

WHICH IS BETTER TO REPLACE SWEAT LOSSES – WATER OR SPORTS DRINKS?

Sports drinks are important during endurance exercise like marathons to help replace fluids and energy. This helps prevent both mental and physical fatigue. If you exercise for more than an hour, a sports drink taken during the workout will provide the energy you need, and if you are exercising for less than an hour, water is generally fine. After a hard workout, you can easily replace carbohydrates and fluids with juices. Due to the fact sports drinks are diluted for rapid absorption, they are a weaker source of carbohydrates than juice, so you need to drink twice as much sports drink (about thirty-two ounces) to get enough carbohydrates about fifty grams (200 calories) every two hours after exercise.

THE TRUTH ABOUT SWEAT

During running, muscles generate heat and lots of it. A typical five-mile run burns about 500 calories, and 70 percent of this heat must exit the body to keep muscle tissue from literally cooking. The body stays cool by producing sweat, the evaporation of which rids your body of unwanted heat, which is roughly 600 calories of heat for every quart of sweat that evaporates. During an hour of running, you can easily lose more than two quarts of sweat.

How much you sweat depends upon several factors. Warm weather and high humidity both increase sweat production. The faster you run, the more heat you generate, so the more you sweat. Sweat rate is also influenced by your fitness level and the sweat glands in a fit body enlarge and increase in number, so you sweat more. All these bodily adjustments create more efficient cooling while you run.

Reference: https://www.thermapparel.com/blog/interesting-facts-about-sweating-breathing-and-the-science-of-cooling-our-bodies

PROTECT YOURSELF FROM DEHYDRATION

An athlete's body needs fluids to function properly. As sweat, fluids cool the skin, blood carries body heat to the skin and as sweat evaporates, the heat escapes. Fluids also thin blood, letting it flow easily through tiny capillaries and carry energizing oxygen to all muscle cells.

When dehydration occurs, blood thickens and moves slowly. Less fluid is available for sweat, so less cooling occurs. When an athlete loses 3 percent of body weight through sweat — or about 4. 5 pounds of a 150-pound athlete — muscular endurance decreases markedly. If the athlete continues to lose fluids, heat cramps will follow and even death could result. Even the performance of the best fit runners will suffer if they are dehydrated.

You can guard against dehydration by making sure you have a fluid replacement plan, especially in hot weather. The hotter it is, the greater the threat of dehydration because athletes sweat more. In the worst conditions, dehydration can occur immediately during a long run. Dehydration can also occur over a few days if the athlete is running a lot and not replacing enough fluid each day. The maximum sweat rate is one to three liters per hour and the maximal gastric emptying rate, which is how fast water leaves the stomach, is one liter per hour. Even under ideal circumstances, dehydration is a threat.

"You are under no obligation to be the same person you were five minutes ago."

— Alan Watts

TIPS FOR TAKING YOUR WORKOUTS TO THE NEXT LEVEL

BENEFITS OF LONGER RUNS

There are people who say, for example, that two fifteen-minute workouts will produce the same amount of weight loss as thirty minutes of continuous exercise and that several shorter workouts lower cholesterol just as much as longer sessions. My belief is that long-run workouts enhance your overall fitness and strength throughout and assist in maintaining your peak of performances throughout the year.

This thought process might make you think that you have no use for longer runs unless you are training for a marathon. This even might lead you to assume that you can split your long runs in half. For example, run six miles in the morning and six miles in the evening and reap the same training effect as doing a continuous twelve-mile run. My belief that this assumption is *not* true.

Long runs have great potential to improve your performance whether you run 5Ks, 10Ks, half marathons or marathons. When you think about it when you focus on performance effects, you will find that a workout lasting thirty-five minutes or more is definitely better than two or more shorter sessions that add up to the same amount of time. Most elite middle-distance runners even incorporate weekly long-run workouts throughout most of the year. During my post-collegiate career, my training partner Steve Scott and I would run nineteen miles together for a Sunday workout.

During a longer workout you recruit more muscle fibers, fire up fat metabolism, and even experience higher heart rates than you would during a shorter effort. Long runs also increase your weekly mileage, boost your maximal aerobic capacity (max V02), and strengthen your leg muscles.

Long runs increase your endurance and your ability to run for long periods without stopping. In closing, a ten-mile run, for example, will give you more fitness than two five-milers.

YOUR PERFORMANCE WILL IMPROVE BY RUNNING LONGER AND FASTER!

Two other approaches to making long runs work for you are the following:

1. Concentrate on intensity – You will improve your fitness much quicker running ten miles at nearly your five-mile training pace. If you run the ten-miler at a slower pace you will not get the maximum benefits.

2. Run at your goal race pace during part of your long run so the stamina gained from a long run is only relevant to the pace used during that run. For example, if you complete twenty miles at an eight-minute per mile pace, you should not have any trouble finishing a marathon at that speed. However, you probably will not do as well if your marathon goal pace is seven-minute miles. In fact, a ten-mile run at seven-minute pace would help you reach your goal more than doing a twenty-miler at a slower pace.

In closing, please do not be so concerned about the specific length of your long runs but instead focus on adding quality to them. You should cover "easy" miles within your long run workouts, and I recommend you run them at between forty-five seconds to ninety seconds per mile slower than your goal race pace. For other long run workouts feel free to add quality miles at goal pace too.

TWO WAYS TO IMPROVE SPEED

There are many ways to get faster, but which are the right ones for you? What everyone needs is a more comprehensive approach that focuses on two key components:

1. Max Vo2 is simply your maximum rate of oxygen use. Max Vo2 goes up as your heart gets stronger and as your leg muscles improve their ability to process oxygen from the blood. Fitness enthusiasts like myself discover that when increasing your max Vo2 it will definitely enable you to run faster and longer at the same effort level. I suggest you can do a max Vo2 building workout every other week.

2. Strength: If you cannot run, you cannot improve. Let's face it, the activity of running is a sport specific training activity. If your goal is to be faster, then you must run. Keep in mind you work off strength to gain speed so that requires incorporating weekly recovery run workouts, one weekly long run throughout the year, and a season of lactate threshold workouts in your regimen. Furthermore, research shows that runners who strength train regularly are injured less often than those who do not emphasize strength. Becoming stronger from the waist down can make you a more powerful, faster runner. I recommend at least twice a week to strengthen the muscles, connective tissues, and ligaments of the legs by doing leg presses, leg curls, heel raises, and toe raises. Improve foot strength by doing strides on a flat grassy area once a week.

DEFINING LACTATE THRESHOLD VELOCITY

Lactate threshold velocity is the running speed beyond which lactate begins to accumulate in the blood. The important thing to remember is that as lactate threshold velocity increases, your race times will improve. This is an essential component in everyone's training plan. Between the years of 1988 to 1996, I had the wonderful privilege to train with former American Record Holder in the one-mile, Steve Scott. I can personally attest that tempo run workouts are the mainstay for success in everyone's distance running training plan.

Athletes often overlook the importance of Lactate Threshold Velocity and its benefits. A classic lactate threshold velocity workout is to run ten-minute intervals at your current 10K pace with five-minute recovery between each interval. This should be done every ten days and if you are a new runner, do two or three repeats per session. More experienced runners should aim for three or four.

I have experienced great results from my athletes with respect to tempo running, so what is the physiological secret behind tempo running? Tempo runs are excellent for developing stamina, confidence, and a sense of pace.

For a beginner my recommendation when doing tempo run workouts is you need to warm up with an easy ten-minute jog, then run for twenty to twenty-five minutes at tempo pace, which is ten to fifteen seconds per mile slower than 10K race pace *or* thirty seconds per mile slower than 5K race pace. For example, if one runs 18:50 for a 5K is 6:05 pace so then you add thirty seconds and tempo pace would be 6:35 mile pace. Finish with a cool-down jog. This workout should not be too exhausting, rather, it should feel comfortably hard.

Tempo run workouts are geared for both the beginner and advanced runners and it took years, but the tempo workouts that Steve Scott and I ran consisted of ten miles at 5:00 pace. It was all relative since our pace was based on the fitness level that we were at during that time. It's common for sub four-minute milers to run their tempo runs at five-minute pace just as it's common for recreational runners to complete their tempo run workouts at a six- or seven-minute pace.

There is a specific psychological benefit to tempo running. Unlike short duration interval style training, tempo runs require you to run hard for relatively long periods which nicely imitates actual racing. Tempo runs raise your lactate threshold velocity, the running speed above which fatigue sets in quickly. As your lactate threshold velocity increases, you'll run at faster speeds without getting tired. In other words, tempo running is an excellent bridge to racing; it requires you to run hard for relatively long periods, and it's recommended you run tempo runs weekly for three months leading up to your highly competitive season. This workout can take a lot out of you so during the seasonal period you are doing it, I recommend doing it once a week.

LACTATE THRESHOLD WORKOUTS EXAMPLES

As discussed, a lactate threshold run is a sustained run of at least twenty minutes or longer at a pace thirty seconds slower than one's own current 5K race pace. By doing this type of training it allows you to maintain your race pace longer and it makes you stronger. Below are some lactate threshold workouts you can do in your own training:

1. **Steppingstone Run:** You run each mile or section of miles faster than the previous run. For example, a ten-mile run can consist of running the first two miles' easy warm-up, then start with a mile at about sixty seconds slower than your current 10K pace. I recommend you then run each successive mile ten seconds faster than the previous one until your last mile is run at current 10K race pace.

2. **Cruise Intervals:** This is a great way for beginning runners to do a lactate threshold workout. Run interval repetitions of 1600 meters, 2400 meters or 3200 meters in length at lactate threshold pace with no more than sixty seconds recovery between reps. Below are three types of intervals you can do at lactate threshold pace:

   > 4 x 1600 meters
   > 3 x 2400 meters
   > 2 x 3200 meters

3. **Lactate Threshold Pace Run:** Consists of completing a twenty to twenty-five-minute run without a break at lactate threshold pace after an appropriate warm-up and followed by an appropriate cool-down.

4. **Marathon Pace Run:** This workout is geared specifically for marathoners whereby you do a thirty-minute warm-up then run six

miles at marathon pace, four miles at lactate threshold pace, and finish with a one-mile warm-down.

5. **10 Mile Run** using the first two miles as a warm-up and I recommend you then alternate between running the next mile at your current 10K pace, then the next sixty seconds, run your next mile at your current 10K pace and back again. Do this until you reach the eight-mile mark and you're finished.

I highly recommend these workouts should occur every seven to fifteen days. You should find that after four to six of these lactate threshold sessions, I believe your strength will show dramatic improvement and with strength your speed improves.

THE BENEFITS OF SPEED TRAINING

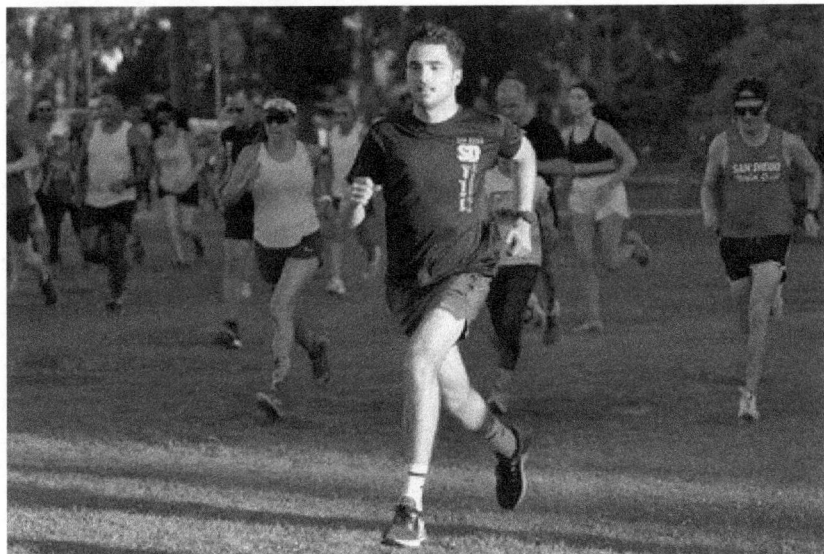

Since the energy demands of long-distance running are predominantly aerobic, sprinting will account for very little of your training time. Nonetheless, speed is a component of all running and an athlete's ability to sprint well at the end of a race often determines the outcome of individual competition. Speed training helps develop sprinting ability, good running mechanics, and physical strength.

During my competitive career as a middle-distance runner that began in high school, continued in college, and went on to compete post-collegiately, I had great success in focusing on speed throughout the year.

Keep in mind that distance runners are generally not sprinters. They need to learn to run fast with distance running mechanics. The fatigue of a 5K or 10K race rarely allows a runner to sprint like a 100-meter runner. Efficient mechanics and an emphasis on stride frequency are the best ways to improve a distance runner's speed.

The preferred method of developing speed for distance runners is to include some speed training within the body of the workout one to two times per week. Adding speed buildups or ten strides before or after continuous runs is one good recommended method.

DEFINITION OF TEMPO INTERVALS (THRESHOLD TRAINING)

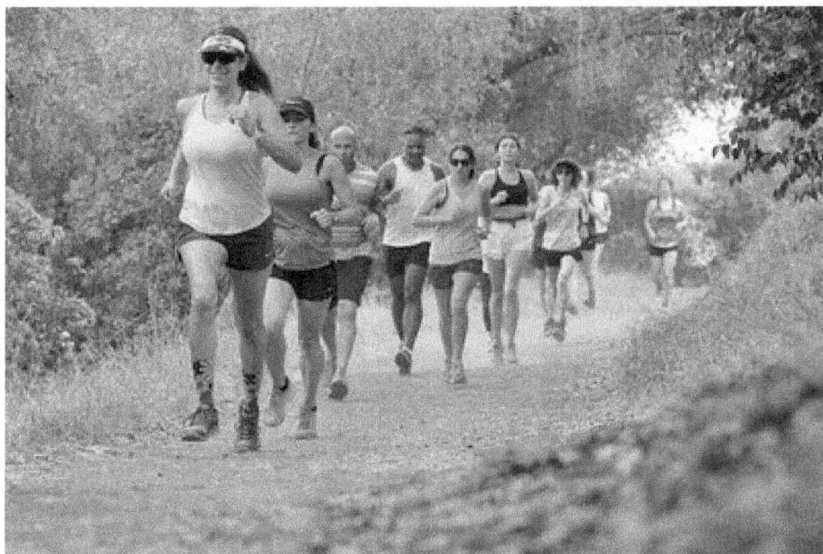

Tempo pace running is designed to maximize aerobic capacity and increase aerobic efficiency. Regular threshold training enables runners to increase pace without suffering from lactate acid accumulation. Athletes should do these runs at a pace that can be maintained for twenty to thirty-five minutes. Tempo runs should be done at a pace that puts the athlete at or slightly above their anaerobic or lactate threshold.

Threshold training can be continuous or segmented. Continuous training, usually called tempo runs, is typically done for twenty to forty minutes at a pace thirty to forty seconds per mile slower than 5K race pace. Warm-up and warm-down running should precede and follow the tempo run.

Segmented threshold training is also referred to as tempo reps or tempo intervals. This training consists of a series of shorter runs lasting anywhere from ninety seconds to eight minutes or 600 meters to 2000 meters with short rest intervals of one minute or less. A tempo rep workout will usually take thirty to forty minutes with recovery included within this workout. One prescribed tempo interval workout that I have seen many of my runners execute with solid results is to run 24 x 200's at a pace thirty seconds slower than one's own current 5K race pace with thirty seconds recovery between each interval.

DEFINITION OF STEADY STATE PACE TRAINING

My own definition of steady pace training is different than lactate threshold training (tempo runs) since in my view these runs are relatively slow, continuous long-distance running where the aerobic system remains in a steady state with energy demands.

Long, steady runs should be done at a pace that can be maintained comfortably for forty to sixty minutes. As for intensity on these runs, try sixty to ninety seconds per mile slower than 5K race pace. A good approximation of this intensity is the talk test. I recommend runners should run at a pace that lets them hold a conversation.

Steady pace training develops aerobic and cardiovascular capacity (Vo2 max), improves muscle capillarity, and enhances the efficiency of energy production. Coaches like myself refer to long, steady state runs as the base or foundation training that precedes more intense tempo runs.

DEFINITION OF SPEED PLAY (FARTLEK TRAINING)

Speed play is the literal translation of the Swedish Word Fartlek. It combines fast and slow running within a continuous run. Different times of fast running are followed by easy recovery running. Ideally, speed play is done over varied terrain, including running over hills. The length of speed bursts and recovery is generally unstructured so that the athlete gains a genuine feeling of playing with speed.

Since the aim of fartlek training is to develop speed in the context of long-distance running, the overall pace should be relatively easy. Only the speed bursts should be done with any intensity. However, speed play is not easy training. In working with my athletes, I recommend speed bouts anywhere between thirty seconds and five minutes. The entire run will last twenty to forty-five minutes. The number of speed bouts depends on their length and the total length of the run. Remember, athletes should recover between each sprint, and it's not intended to be high lactate training.

In my experience with coaching runners, they tend to need some structure to reap the benefits of fartlek workouts. Fartlek training is excellent mode of training that avoids the hard terrain of a track.

As a competitor myself I found fartlek training a great substitute if running around a track was not possible or I needed a break from the rigors of running around a track.

THE DEFINITION OF INTERVAL TRAINING

Interval training is a frequently misunderstood concept. Most coaches use the terms interval and repetition interchangeably, but they are very different types of training. A repetition is a single unit of running. An interval is the recovery period that follows individual bouts of running.

In repetition training, the objective is to run specific distances at race pace with a relatively complete recovery. With interval training, the goal is to run specific distances with incomplete recovery so that the athlete trains with elevated blood lactate.

Interval training enhances a runner's ability to tolerate and produce lactic acid; while interval training does help raise the lactate threshold it is primarily anaerobic. High lactate training is most specific to long distance runners.

The duration of each run in an interval session is typically fifteen to ninety seconds or 100 to 600 meters. The recovery ratio should be between 1:1 and 2:1, run to recovery. Interval training should be done faster than race pace. The intention of these workouts is to produce lactic acid by forcing your athletes to run the last portion of each repetition anaerobically.

Generally, interval training is intense, demanding, and painful. I recommend not to schedule more than two sessions during any single week of training. Some athletes might require two to three days of easy workouts to recover fully from a hard interval session.

RECOVERY TIME BETWEEN INTERVALS

The duration of recovery between intervals should be long enough to allow your heart rate to go down to 65 percent of maximum heart rate. If you reduce the recovery too short, you'll likely need to shorten the workout, and will not obtain as great a training stimulus. A shortened recovery might mean that you will have to run subsequent intervals too anaerobically which is not the meaning of V02 max workouts. If your recovery is too long, the training stimulus will also be reduced.

The optimal amount of recovery between intervals depends on the length of the intervals you are running. As a general guideline, the rest between intervals should be from 50 percent to 90 percent of the amount of time it takes to run the interval. For example, if one of my athletes runs 1,200-meter repeats in 4:30 (6:00 mile pace), their recovery jog should last 50 percent to 90 percent of this time or between 2:15 and 4:00.

I recommend that during the time between intervals you need to resist the temptation to stand bent over with your hands on your knees. As strange as it might sound, research has shown that you recover the quickest when you easy jog during your recovery, because doing so helps to clear lactic acid from your blood.

THE BENEFITS TO REPETITION TRAINING & VALUE OF TRAINING AT RACE PACE

The purpose of repetition training is to increase aerobic efficiency thereby raising the lactate threshold in relation to Vo2 max. Such training allows a runner to train at Vo2 max, above the threshold level for periods longer than can be sustained in a race. Repetitions also help the athlete develop pace and rhythm.

Repetitions should be from one to six minutes long or distances of 400 to 1600 meters. Pace will vary according to distance. Repetitions that total more than 5000 meters should be done at current race pace. The rest period should provide slightly less than complete recovery and a 1:2 run to recovery ratio is recommended. The workout should total twenty to twenty-five minutes of running.

At times all runners have concerns in their workout routine and training flaws that prevent them from performing at their absolute best. One of the most common is the failure to do some training at actual race pace.

A typical runner hoping to run a forty-minute 10K (6:26 per mile) does long training runs at eight-minute pace, tries a few upbeat workouts at seven-minute pace, and sprints through some eighty-second 400s on the track. Ironically, on race day, this runner expects to cruise through a 10K at 6:26 pace, even though he or she has not practiced it once during training.

In my humble opinion, this will not work, and you should not do all of your training at slower or faster than race pace. In addition to improving performance times, practicing race pace can assist you in being more of a consistently successful runner. With no proper sense of pace, many competitive runners burst from the starting line like sprinters.

Unfortunately, this excess early speed produces a massive rise in blood lactic acid, which can slow you down during the remainder of the race.

Recent research suggests that runners who build up high levels of lactate early in a race tend to run their 5K or 10K races slower than usual.

BENEFITS OF A GOOD POSTURE WHILE RUNNING

The question arises of whether it is too late to change your running style. The answer is no, and a strong upright carriage is one of the most important aspects of running because so many things follow from it. Below are some benefits of a good posture while running:

1. **You'll move as one:** When your body is upright, you'll move forward as one unit with all your muscles working together. Your muscles will not be wasting energy and maintaining balance is important.

2. **You'll run more easily:** Upright posture helps keep the whole body in proper alignment. When you're in proper alignment, you'll generate maximum power, which reduces the effort required to run at any pace.

3. **You'll increase speed more easily:** An upright body allows your legs to extend maximally with no extra effort. With this kind of extension, you'll be able to shift gears more easily because you're already in the proper biomechanical position.

4. **You'll get injured less:** When you reduce inefficient leanings and extraneous motions your muscles and tendons will spend less time correcting these problems. Therefore, they'll be less likely to succumb to overuse injury.

5. **You'll breathe easier:** When you're upright, you'll get maximum breathing capacity from your lungs. A forward lean makes it tougher for you to fill your lungs and use your diaphragm properly. Stronger, deeper breathing allows you to obtain more oxygen in and out of the lungs.

6.   **You'll cut down on side stiches:** By incorporating better breathing good posture makes it less likely that you'll develop stiches.

Please be patient and diligent when working on your posture since it takes time to see some notable improvement. For me personally it was years before I ran with good form that translated to running fast times and being a sub four-minute miler.

GOOD RUNNING POSTURE TRANSLATES TO FASTER PERFORMANCES

Having observed thousands of runners over the years I have seen that those who lean too far forward normally cut approximately an inch from each stride. In essence, they do this in order to maintain balance. An inch per stride might not sound like much, but it works out to almost 1000 feet in a 10K and about 4000 feet over the course of a marathon. At ten-minute per mile pace, this means a person who stays upright would finish the marathon more than seven minutes faster and with no extra effort.

Strengthening your postural muscles will help you run upright from the beginning of your run. Furthermore, once you're stronger it becomes less likely that you will slip out of position when fatigue sets in. If you think bad posture is a serious problem for you, I recommend you talk to your doctor about it. He or she can refer you to a physical therapist or strength trainer who will help you get back into shape with a specific plan geared to your needs.

One exercise I suggest is arm running, whereby to balance abdominal strength, you need to build up your back and sides too. A great way to do this is by *Arm Running with hand-held weights*. If you don't have dumbbells, you can always use water-filled plastic jugs. To do this exercise, stand erect, hold onto the weights, and begin moving your arms as you do during running, while keeping your feet firmly planted. You might want to glance at a mirror while you do this, so you'll be sure to stay in the proper posture. As with running, keep your elbows bent at roughly 90 degrees as you pump your arms. Continue until fatigue sets in and I recommend you try to do this exercise every other day.

WAYS TO IMPROVE POSTURE WHILE RUNNING

Before I share some ways to improve posture, you might want to get a better idea of how you're doing in this department. I recommend having a friend or family member videotape your running from the side. If you don't have access to a video recorder or even an iPhone, have someone stand and watch you closely as you run. Are you leaning too far forward? Too far backward? Are your shoulders hunched? Is your head slung forward? Once you have something to work with it's time to start perfecting your posture.

I have learned over the years, when I occasionally have trouble straightening up on a run, I envision myself being suspended by a string attached to the top of my head. As I hang there, gravity efficiently aligns my head, torso, and pelvis. I complete the vision by imagining my feet lightly touching down as the legs go through their smooth-running circuit.

This puppet visualization will help you stay upright and light on your feet, both of which will allow you to conserve energy and run more efficiently. Another visualization technique you might try is to imagine that you have a pulley attached to the center of your breastbone. The other end of the pulley is attached by a rope to the top of a low building one block away. As you run, imagine that the rope is pulling you toward the top of the building. This will help lift your chest and it's important to not lean forward as you want your whole chest leading the way forward.

Good body alignment is essential, in fact, it is critical in an exercise program. Our bodies are meant to move. However, if we exercise incorrectly, we may very well create imbalances in our body. Some muscle groups are then working harder than they should, not allowing other muscle groups to do their job. These imbalances eventually can be seen as chronic aches and injuries.

Gravity is always with us so, to function effortlessly, good posture is critical. The center of gravity of our body lies just at the lumbar-sacral articulation. The sacrum is the structural and energy center of the body, where all of the mechanical movements of the body are centered. Forces on the body are directly transmitted to this point. Proper sacrum alignment and balance are critical to exercising with maximum safety and efficiency. Since people often function in poor alignment, it is easy to see why so many suffer from chronic back pain.

In many cases, knee problems are related directly to the alignment of the ankle, knee, and hip joints; similarly, elbow problems can be related to the alignment of the wrist, elbow, and shoulder joints.

I recommend you should observe your posture and alignment. Does one foot usually turn out when you're just standing around? Do your shoulders hunch forward throughout the day? Ask a friend to analyze your posture. A stretching and strengthening program will help you achieve good alignment. Remember, good posture radiates youthfulness, strength, and an enthusiastic, positive outlook on life.

RUNNING ON SAND

Without question, running on sand is frustrating; you feel like a dying snail. The important thing to remember is that everyone else feels the same too. Physically, dig the front of your foot into the sand by landing toe first, and angle forward to a point that almost feels like you will tip over.

With running in sand, attempt to pick a spot on the beach where the sand is the hardest, usually the wet sand closer to the waves. Be careful not to get your shoes all wet and heavy though and be aware of the angle of the sand since repetitive running at that surface may lead to stress on the hip region of your body. This is problematic and causes IT band syndrome and tight piriformis injuries. Try not to roll an ankle or lose time worrying about staying balanced, and I also recommend choosing a little heavier shoe with a wider sole when running in sand especially if you are accustomed to running on this type of surface frequently. Obviously, living by the beach in San Diego provides plenty of opportunities for fitness enthusiasts to run on sand and the fondest memories of my adolescence were running at the beach on the sand.

HELPFUL TIPS TO UPHILL RUNNING

Every summer for the past thirty-seven years I always prescribed ten weeks of uphill running workouts with the San Diego Track Club on Tuesday nights. As you start running up hills shorten your stride and concentrate on lifting your knees and landing more toward the front of your foot. You lean slightly forward but keep your back straight, your hips in, your chest out and your head up. Pump your arms forward and downward and not across your body.

It's important you breathe from the belly and stay relaxed. The key to uphill running form is to learn to switch naturally into an efficient power gear, the same way you would switch gears when you drive your car up a steep hill.

Resist the temptation to look all the way to the top of the hill. You might be intimidated by how far away the top appears, so I recommend you pick a landmark such as a car, house, fire hydrant or telephone pole. Imagine that a rope is tied to a runner or object in front of you and that you can pull yourself up the hill into small manageable pieces. By doing it this way you can make even an enormous incline seem relatively easy.

Do not try to maintain the same pace you were running on the flat as this will only exhaust you and leave you depleted later in your run. If necessary, take baby steps and try to keep the same turnover rhythm as on the flat. Your posture should be upright so don't lean forward or back. Head, shoulders, and hips should form a straight line over the feet. Keep your feet low to the ground and if your breathing begins to quicken this means you're either going too fast, over striding or bounding too far off the ground.

If the hill is long and/or the grade increases, my recommendation is to keep shortening your stride to maintain a smooth and efficient breathing pattern. It's always recommended you run through the top of the hill and do not immediately slow down or pull back your effort. Rather, accelerate gradually into the downhill as gravity is now on your side.

When running uphill don't worry if you're slowing down going up, just reduce stride length accordingly, and as you shorten your stride, keep your feet directly under your body.

RUNNING HILLS DOESN'T HAVE TO BE INTIMIDATING

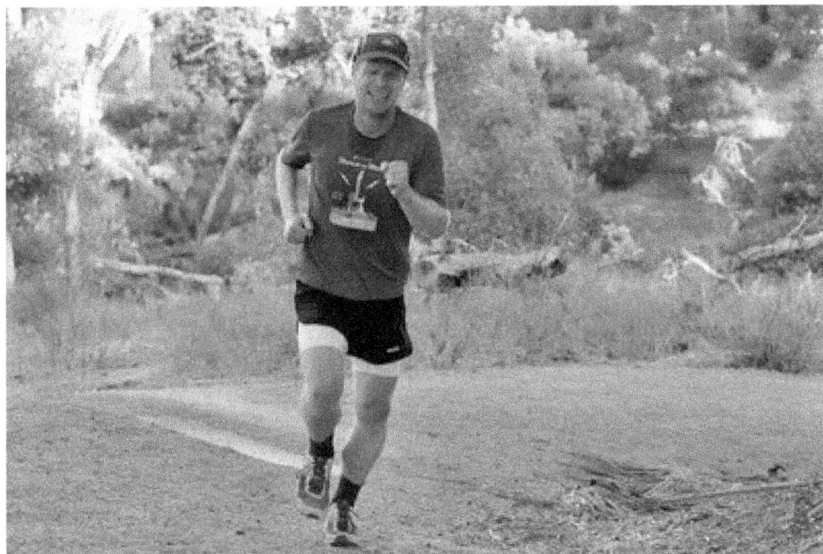

For years, hill training was always built into my routine during the fall season in preparation of racing the one mile during the spring's track season. Hills do not have to hurt, and they don't have to be overwhelming. There are techniques you can learn that will make hill running easier. By shortening your stride and running with a light rhythm you can feel nearly as good running uphill as you do on flat ground. With relaxed, controlled strides you will also be able to run down hills without thrashing your legs. Hills are great for teaching rhythm, one of the most overlooked and crucial aspects of distance running, and keep in mind if you let hills break up your rhythm, you will slow down drastically. Furthermore, if you make the proper adjustments to maintain cadence you will improve the performance on hills.

Whether you are going up or down hills I recommend you try to maintain the same level of effort and breathing rate that you use on flat ground. Don't worry if you're slowing down running uphill so just reduce stride length accordingly. You continue to shorten your stride when the hill is steeper and extend to normal as the hill eases all the while maintaining steady effort and breathing.

It's a wonderful revelation when one realizes there is a stride short enough to give you control over the steepest of hills. As you shorten your stride and keep your feet directly under your body you will gain efficiency needed to be successful on hills. With this efficiency comes momentum and confidence.

UPHILL RUNNING TECHNIQUE AND COMMON PROBLEMS EXPERIENCED

As already pointed out, hills are great for teaching rhythm, one of the most overlooked and crucial aspects of distance running. Common problems athletes face and the reasons for these problems on running uphill are listed below:

1. Breathing too rapidly is caused by over striding or bounding too high.

2. Tight leg muscles result in over striding.

3. Tight or sore lower back is caused by leaning too far forward.

4. Shoulders and arms tired and sore results in too much arm swing or arms too far forward.

What has already been pointed out already, you need to remember what's critical when running up hills is to reduce the stride length but maintain the same stride rhythm and breathing rate.

DOWNHILL RUNNING TECHNIQUE

Downhill running can be your best friend or your worst enemy. If you have good downhill running technique, you will benefit from gravity to increase your speed and cover more ground. However, if you have bad downhill running technique, you risk too much pounding on your feet, tightening your hamstrings, and overusing your quadriceps. Learn how to run downhill like an elite runner!

First – what NOT to do: While it might seem contradictory, avoid leaning too far forward and catching too much air. Doing this will cause over striding, which leads to stress on your body and lack of stability and speed management. Being out of control uses extra energy, negating the benefits of the downhill. You are essentially fighting yourself.

What TO do: Relax and don't over stride. Avoid catching too much air by keeping your feet low to the ground. Doing this will provide you with more control. Touch lightly with each step and allow the steepness of the hill to dictate your stride. As you focus on keeping your feet low to the ground, you should feel as if your stride is shorter. Don't let this fool you. As a result of running downhill, your stride is covering more ground than you think! The key here is to keep low to the ground, avoid over striding, stay light on your feet, and relax. The momentum you gain going downhill is a wonderful source of energy as you continue your run to level terrain or to another hill.

DOWNHILL RUNNING TECHNIQUE AND COMMON PROBLEMS EXPERIENCED

I'm often asked what the proper downhill running technique should be for success. For starters, it is recommended that you increase stride rhythm in response to the downslope, but do not over stride. Also, always keep feet low to the ground.

Shown below are common downhill running problems that athletes face:

- Over striding can cause tight hamstrings and sore shins.
- Overstriding can also force quadriceps to work too hard, risking injury.
- Running too fast can cause flailing arms and loss of rhythm.
- Leaning back (to avoid falling forward) can cause lower back pain.

Overall, it is recommended to stay as relaxed as possible when running downhill. Staying relaxed will help you avoid common downhill challenges.

USING HILL TRAINING TO IMPROVE SPEED!

Downhill running is a method of speed-assisted training that uses gravity to increase stride frequency. Speed-assisted training is primarily neurological training that prompts the nervous system to spend impulses to activate muscle activity much more quickly than normal.

Using downhill running to better extend this kind of neurological/ physiological training benefit is applicable for middle- and long-distance runners. A moderate downhill slope of forty to a hundred meters is an ideal venue for speed training. A training sequence of assist-resist-assist has been shown to be the most effective method for stimulating neurological activity at maximum speeds. This translates to doing four to six reps of forty to one hundred meters of downhill sprinting followed by four to six reps of sprinting the same distance uphill, followed by four to six more downhill repetitions.

It's recommended you incorporate a walking recovery back up or down the hill with an additional two to five-minute recovery between sets. The training session should end at any point when you can no longer maintain good running mechanics or when the return walks no longer provide sufficient recovery between reps.

HILL WORKOUTS ARE YOUR FRIENDS

Below are four hill workouts where one can be incorporated each week in your training. These hill workouts have been prescribed for the San Diego Track Club runners to complete over the years.

1. **Repeats** are approached by finding a hill that's a 4 percent to 10 percent grade and takes approximately ninety seconds to run. You'll run the hill from six to ten times in the workout, depending on how far along you are in your training. Before you run the hill, you'll need to do a fifteen to twenty-minute warm-up. Once you're well warmed up, stretch for a few minutes and follow the stretching with six 100-meter strides. Remember that, when you're running up the hill, you should shorten your stride, lift your knees, and lean forward slightly. The recovery is the time required to run back down. As soon as you reach the bottom, you'll start back up again. Finish the workout with an easy twenty-minute jog.

2. **Hill Circuits:** Find a location where you can run a succession of hills for forty-five minutes to one hour. An ideal route would be one with three to five hills that takes thirty minutes to run. You can run out for thirty minutes, then turn around and run back the same set of hills. You'll run each hill hard, then do an easy jog to the next one.

3. **Hill Circuits Concentrating on Running Form:** This can be a difficult workout to do but, if you do it once every other week or so, you'll reap tremendous benefits. Run the same set of hills as in the hill circuit's workout. Concentrate on running a steady pace between the hills instead of easy jogging. You'll emphasize pace — not on the hill but running from hill to hill. Use the hills to concentrate on your running form. Don't try to run hard on the way up the hill but instead slow down and think about how you're running. Then, when

you crest the top of the hill, take five to fifteen quick steps off the top of the hill and get back into the steady pace you'll maintain on the flats until you reach the next hill. The key to the success of this workout is that, when you do it, you'll never quite feel you've had a full recovery. Besides this workout making you stronger, this workout will teach you how to effectively race hills. Too often runners will charge up a hill in a race, slow down significantly at the top, and then end up being passed because they've run out of gas and need to recover. Don't let it happen to you! Do this workout regularly and you'll certainly blow your competition away.

4. **Three Minute Steady-State** is a great workout for raising your lactate threshold velocity (the speed above which fatigue sets in quickly). Identify a hill that will take you approximately twenty-five minutes to run from bottom to top. Using your heart rate monitor, run up the hill/mountain hard until you reach 80 percent to 85 percent of your maximum heart rate. Maintain that rate for three minutes. You'll then do a one-minute recovery jog, still heading uphill. Continue alternating three minutes hard with one minute easy until you've reached the top of the hill or until you've run for twenty-five minutes.

DEFINING VO2 MAX

Most serious runners and certainly running coaches know that a high VO2 max is important for good racing. In 5K and 10K distances it's the most important physiological attribute in determining your success and it's of equal importance to a high lactate threshold. VO2 max also contributes significantly to your finishing time in the marathon. Most runners don't know what VO2 max is so provided is the simplistic definition for VO2 max.

Runners with a high VO2 max have a plumbing system if you will that allows them to pump large amounts of oxygen-rich blood to working muscles. With training, you can maximize the size of your pump and the quantity of blood that it transports. Specifically, your VO2 max is the maximal amount of oxygen that your heart can pump to your muscles and that your muscles can then use to produce energy. It's the product of your heart rate times the amount of blood pumped per beat times the proportion of oxygen extracted from the blood and used by your muscles.

More precisely your VO2 max is important because it determines your aerobic capacity so the higher your VO2 max, the greater your ability to produce energy aerobically. With everything being the same the more energy you can produce aerobically, the faster a pace you can maintain.

HOW TO DETERMINE YOUR VO2 MAX?

Often, I share this important information with my Kinesiology students at San Diego City College, along with the distance runners I coach with the San Diego Track Club. The greatest stimulus to improving VO2 max comes by training at an intensity that requires 95 percent to 100 percent of your current VO2 max. Questions come up with respect to the methods used for determining VO2 max. Below are four options.

You can find out by having your VO2 max measured at an exercise physiology lab and in this test, you start running slowly then the speed or incline of the treadmill is increased every few minutes until you cannot keep up. The test usually takes about ten to fifteen minutes.

If you don't have access to a lab, you can make an educated guess of your VO2 max running pace based on your racing times. Your running speed at 95 percent to 100 percent of your VO2 max should be about your 3000-meter to 5000-meter race pace. Doing a portion of your training at this pace will provide the greatest stimulus to improving your VO2 max. You will stress your cardiovascular system to its limit, which will help to increase your stroke volume and improve your ability to extract oxygen from the blood.

You can also estimate the appropriate intensity for VO2 max training based on your heart rate. VO2 max training pace coincides with approximately 95 percent to 100 percent of your maximal heart rate. You should keep your heart rate several beats under your maximum during this type of training. Otherwise, you'll work too intensely which will shorten the workout and tend to provide less stimulus to improve VO2 max. Your body can positively respond to only a limited amount of training at VO2 max intensity before you break down. Ideally, you'll find the correct balance in terms of the volume of training per VO2 max workout and how frequently you do these workouts, so that you train at V02 max intensity often enough to improve but avoid becoming over-trained.

Finally, a less scientific way to determine V02 max that would provide a close measurement but not exact one is to run 10 x 200-yard hills with a 4 percent incline and recovery would be to jog back down the hill you just ran. After the tenth and final hill repeat simply take your pulse and surprisingly your V02 max measurement can be close enough to an actual measured one in the physiology lab.

RECOMMENDED VOLUME AND FREQUENCY FOR VO2 MAX WORKOUTS

Many experts agree that you will improve VO2 max most rapidly by running 2.5 miles to six miles of intervals per workout. The optimal volume within that range depends on your training history. If you run less than 2.5 miles of intervals, you will still provide a training stimulus, but your rate of improvement will be slower. If you try to run more than six miles of intervals at this intensity, then you will most likely either not be able to maintain the appropriate pace for the entire time or will become so tired from the workout that you will not recover quickly enough for your next workout. For most runners, sessions of three to four miles of intervals provide the most effective balance.

The best way to improve your VO2 max quickly is by running one high volume workout at 95 percent to 100 percent of VO2 max per week. Depending on the distance you will be racing and the number of weeks until your goal race, it may be beneficial to complete a second lower VO2 max workout during certain weeks.

RECOMMENDED DURATION FOR VO2 MAX WORKOUTS

It's understood by most running experts that your greatest gains in VO2 max can be made by running repetitions of two to six minutes' duration. For most runners, this means intervals of approximately 600 meters to one mile. Besides going to a track, you can also do your VO2 max workouts running on a golf course. The greatest stimulus to improve aerobic capacity is getting your cardiovascular system up to 95 percent to 100 percent of VO2 max and maintaining it in that range for as long as possible during the workout.

Short intervals are not nearly as effective in providing this stimulus because you don't accumulate enough time in the optimal intensity range. For example, if you run 400 meter repeats it will be easy to hold VO2 max pace, but you will only be at pace for a short time during each interval. As a result, you will have to run lots of 400s to provide much stimulus to improve your VO2 max. On the other hand, if you run mile repeats at the correct pace, your cardiovascular system will be at 95 percent to 100 percent of VO2 max for several minutes during each interval and during the workout you will accumulate more time at the most effective training intensity.

As a coach I like prescribing the 1200-meter distance and executing repeats at the correct pace your cardiovascular system will be at 95 percent to 100 percent of VO2 max for several minutes during each interval and during the workout, you will accumulate more time at the most effective training intensity.

VOLUME OF TRAINING PER VO2 MAX WORKOUT

As already shared in another fitness tip but it's worth repeating, you'll improve V02 max most rapidly by running 2.5 to six miles or 4000 to 9600 meters of intervals per workout. The optimal volume within that range depends on your training history.

If you run less than 2.5 miles of intervals, you'll still provide a training stimulus, but your rate of improvement will be slower. If you try to run more than six miles of intervals at this intensity, you'll most likely either not be able to maintain the appropriate pace for the entire time or will become so worn out from the workout that you won't recover quickly enough for your next workout. In my experience for most runners, sessions of three to five miles of intervals provide the most effective balance.

SPEED OF INTERVALS FOR VO2 MAX WORKOUTS

Most running coaches would agree that if you run slower than 95 percent to 100 percent of your VO2 max, then you're heading toward lactate threshold training. Lactate threshold training is valuable but your VO2 max workouts are not the place to do it. On the other hand, if you run your intervals faster than the 95 percent to 100 percent of VO2 max training range, you will not provide as great a stimulus to improve your VO2 max pace; you use your anaerobic system, meaning you're improving the wrong area. You might think that the anaerobic system is just as important as the aerobic system, and it is if you're racing 800 meters. If you are racing 5000 meters or farther, the anaerobic system is primarily used only for the finishing part of the race. If you've trained aerobically, while equally talented runners have trained anaerobically, you'll be so far ahead going into your finishing kick that you won't have to worry about their finishing speed.

I believe the other reason that running your intervals too fast provides less stimulus to improve VO2 max is that you simply cannot do as much volume. Remember, the total amount of time accumulated at minutes of work, of which perhaps six minutes were at the most effective intensity to improve VO2 max. However, if you run five repetitions of 1200 meters at your 5K race pace and that means running your repeats in 4:00 for example, you will have completed twenty minutes of hard running, almost all of which is at the appropriate intensity to stimulate improvements in your VO2 max.

My goal as a coach when prescribing these types of workouts is for the workout to end with the athlete feeling they can complete one more interval if it was to be prescribed. By incorporating this approach this will reduce the risk of overtraining in workouts before an upcoming race event.

THE VO2 MAX WORKOUT DESIGN

VO2 max workouts can be categorized into two basic steps:

1. Workouts in which the distance of the interval is constant.
2. Workouts in which they are varied.

Many runners vary the length of intervals within a workout to make the workout easier mentally and this is especially true when it applies to self-coached runners who have done the same and they run ladder workouts that consist of one interval each at a variety of distances on the way up and down the ladder.

Athletes psyche themselves up by saying, "Just one-mile repeat then each one gets shorter on the way down" and in my opinion this approach can be counterproductive because an important element of training as set of intervals of the same length is recommended, because it allows you to learn what it feels like to maintain speed which fatigue increases; therefore, stimulates more closely day of race conditions.

There are times when varying the length of the intervals can be beneficial if you want to run some shorter intervals at the end of the workout to improve your finishing kick of a race.

MOTIVATION IN THE WEIGHT ROOM IS CRITICAL

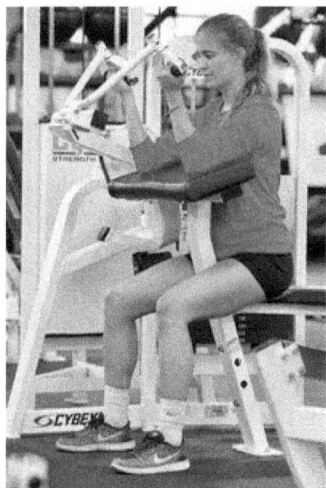

As a Kinesiology Professor at San Diego City College, one of our most popular exercise classes we offer every semester is Fundamentals of Weight Training and this is a class I have personally taught for over thirty years. This class is very popular, and the level of motivation is high. There are four basic areas of motivation in the weight room for athletes, as follows:

1. **Education:** Athletes need to understand the positive aspects of a strength training program and reasons why a program is structured the way it is moving forward. It's important to see the benefits you will receive and correlate what is done in the weight room to how it affects the sport of running. It's important to realize that a stronger athlete is less susceptible to injury.

2. **Organized Program:** A well-organized program produces results and positive results are the best motivation an athlete can receive. A well-prepared, well-structured program gives you confidence and encourages you to give it your all, and poor organization adds doubts in athlete's minds and reduces the credibility of the program. Athletes need a thorough plan and after each workout, these athletes should leave the weight room feeling another step closer to reaching their goals.

3. **Recognition:** Being recognized for one's own effort is important, and this can be done every day with a small compliment. A few simple words to acknowledge something achieved in a previous exercise means a lot to athletes.

4. **Individualized Workouts:** All athletes are different and progress at their own pace. Some are more gifted and get stronger before others. This is why a designed program is critical in assisting athletes to reach their fullest potential. Please do not make the mistake of generalizing the workouts whereby you lift the same amount of weight and do the same exercises multiple times. In this situation some athletes are undertraining while others are overtraining. In both of these cases athletes lose interest in the program and reduce their performance.

A POSITIVE ENVIRONMENT IS A MOTIVATOR IN THE WEIGHT ROOM

Athletes will benefit from being in a positive environment that is conducive to training. Furthermore, I have always believed the greatest motivation for exercise is enjoyment. I say find your joy! Below are four simple guidelines to look for when exercising in a weight room.

1. The weight room needs to be clean.

2. Any unusable equipment must be repaired as quickly as possible.

3. Look for the highest quality equipment when selecting a weight room to work out in.

4. Personal trainers need to be excited about strength training, so enthusiasm is contagious. It's important certified personal trainers have genuine enthusiasm and expect you to stay with the program.

Strength training requires athletes to work constantly at a high level. Without motivation many athletes would not stay with it. Motivation makes a weight training program interesting and exciting, creating in the athlete the desire to improve, excel and reach their ultimate goals. You might agree with my own definition of empowering someone to take action. Motivation is painting a pretty picture and the athlete buys into that pretty picture.

ALTERNATE ENERGY SOURCES

Over the past twenty-five years, I have overseen a full and half marathon training program in San Diego, so every Saturday a few hundred runners gather to run longer distance miles preparing for their choice endurance event. At these run workouts my team would provide water stations every two to three miles where we would offer fluids for the runners to consume. Subsequently, the possibilities of energizing alternatives to regular food are seemingly endless — energy bars, drinks, and even packets of GU. But deciding which product to buy and when to use it can be so overwhelming that you could end up with an empty stomach. Here's all you need to know about high-energy consumption.

What are fluid replacement drinks? They simply are water, simple sugars (i.e., sucrose, glucose, and fructose), and a small number of electrolytes and flavorings. They're available in a variety of flavors and most have fifty to 100 calories and fourteen to twenty-five grams of carbohydrates per eight-ounce serving.

Sports drinks are designed to maximize fluid absorption and provide energizing carbohydrates for performance enhancement. If you like their taste, you're likely to drink more and stay better hydrated than you would with water.

Some of the sports drinks are Gatorade, PowerAde, Allsport. and Cytomax and there are about ten to fifteen others on the market too. Due to hydration being the key to staying energized and there are minimal nutritional differences between most brands of sport drinks, choose the one you find most enjoyable to taste. Whichever brand you choose, drink four to eight ounces every fifteen to twenty minutes during exercise. Best results for most athletes are those who exercise for more than an hour at a time.

HIKING TRAILS IS A GREAT SUBSTITUTE TO RUNNING

Prior to successfully reaching the top of the highest mountain in Africa, Mount Kilimanjaro in 2001, and the highest mountain in mainland Europe, Mount Blanc in 2008, as an alternative to running, I found hiking trails a wonderful substitute to exercise. Trekking up and down terrain while carrying a backpack is weight-bearing exercise that builds bones in addition to burning calories. Before you go hiking one needs to become familiar with the hiking area and know where you are going. Be sure to choose hikes you can physically manage. Below are a few healthy safety tips:

1. Tell a friend or family member about your plans and when you intend to return.

2. Pack enough food for a meal. Some good choices are energy bars, granola, trail mix, and dried fruit.

3. Be sure to bring the essentials, including a basic first aid kit, map, compass, pocketknife, lightweight flashlight, whistle or flare, and waterproof matches.

4. Dress in layers for comfort. Wear sunglasses and a hat or visor and always wear sunscreen.

5. Start out slowly and gradually increase your speed.

6. Stop frequently to rest since tired muscles can lead to injuries as the hike progresses.

7. Use only marked trails.

8. Bring plenty of water including one to two quarts per day to keep hydrated. Be sure to include some electrolyte drinks too.

ANSWERS TO CROSS COUNTRY RUNNING QUESTIONS

I often encourage runners who race one marathon to the next on roads during the year to think about diversifying their running events and take up Cross Country running. Any runner can benefit from the challenges, variety, and injury preventing qualities of trail running. Hitting the trail once or twice a week will make you stronger, improve concentration, and may enliven a training program that's become routine.

Find a suitable course: If you're at a loss, check out local parks, college campuses, the areas around golf courses. Contact running clubs, track and cross-country teams for tips. Try not to run after dark and if you plan to run alone, do so only if you're certain an area is safe. You might want a water bottle.

As for shoes, companies make trail running shoes which have sturdier soles and more durable uppers than road running shoes. Any stable supportive shoe will work. Don't wear cleats, which can snag on roots. Avoid super muddy trails but get used to the idea of getting dirty.

As for running itself, plan to take it easy at first; nothing faster than a jogging pace or longer than about twenty minutes until you've gotten the lay of the land. You may even want to walk a course before jogging it. Enjoy your surroundings and don't get so distracted that you fall. Shorten your stride, lift your knees, and land on the balls of your feet going uphill. On downhills relax and flow landing heel-toe but without pounding on your heels. Have fun as being on trails always feels like a joyful and playful activity.

BENEFITS OF CROSS-COUNTRY TRAIL RUNNING

Cross Country season generally occurs during the fall and it's that time one needs to hit the trails. You may associate training on trails solely with the cross-country crowd. While it's true that off-road running is the mainstay of cross-country training, it can benefit runners of all types. Trail running can add variety, beauty, and new challenges to your training.

As a former intercollegiate cross-country runner, I can attest that the sport is gentle on your knees, it can be done alone or with a group, its accessible just about anywhere, and perhaps best of all, trail running is fun. Trails serve primarily as a means of recovering from speed workouts as the soft surfaces are more forgiving than the roads. In addition, the up and down, the unevenness, the turns, make you use all different muscles. You develop dexterity, balance, and a sense that you can handle challenges. Any runner can benefit from the challenges, variety, and injury-preventing qualities of trail running. Hitting the trails once or twice a week will make you stronger, improve concentration, and may enliven a training program that has become routine.

TRAIL RUNNING SAFETY TIPS

Below are two important preventative safety tips you need to implement when running on trails:

1. **Crash Landings:** You cannot consider yourself a trail runner until you have a few more scars on your body. Falling goes with the territory in technical trail running, even if you're not prone to clumsiness. Usually falls happen so fast, they can't be avoided, and you can avoid a broken collarbone or a concussion by rolling into the fall or trying to brace your fall with an extended arm. It's recommended you be careful and look three steps ahead of where your feet are landing.

2. **Running After Dark:** Running at night on dark trails can be mystical, but only if you have a lightweight headlamp or hand-held light powerful enough to light up the trail. Many low-intensity lights will cast a dim light that offers a blurry view of the rough trail in front of you and that can lead to tripping over hidden obstacles. It's recommended you look for a headlamp with at least five small LEDs. The important thing to remember is to go slow and try not to be overconfident when running in the dark.

TIPS TO TRAIL RUNNING

No two trails are the same, and some trails are hilly or flat or are full of obstacles. Running rugged trails requires some additional skills so provided are two tips that will assist you in approaching effective trail running.

1. **Choose your shoes carefully:** Trail shoes offer greater protection from potential hazards on the trails including a wide, reinforced toe box that helps keep your toes out of harm's way. It's recommended you look for a shoe that offers enough protection and a good amount of agility without being too heavy.

2. **Running Uphill:** When you run uphill rely on your arm swing to maintain your momentum while also shortening your stride and backing off your pace. It's recommended by taking smaller steps, you can maintain your cadence and rhythm without putting yourself into anaerobic trouble. If the trail gets too steep to run, don't feel bad about walking. Many elite athletes will walk steep hills of trail races. With respect to trail running, it's much more efficient at certain times by walking than running.

TRAIL RUNNING TECHNIQUES

Running on trails can definitely present challenges. Below are two additional tips for effective and safe trail running.

1. Learning to run through trails requires additional skills than running on other terrains. It takes practice and the first skill is learning to look three or four steps ahead of where your feet are landing. If you look at your feet, you'll see where they're going to land, but you'll likely trip over something you're not anticipating. By looking ahead, your brain will take a mental picture of the trail and plan your foot placements accordingly. Once you get accustomed to it, it will become second nature and you'll find that you're looking seven or eight strides ahead of your feet.

2. Running down a steep slope can be difficult on smooth terrain. On a rocky trail, it can be terrifying. Until you become proficient at it, keep your speed in check and lean slightly backward, looking just ahead of your feet as they hit the trail. Start down a slope with your elbows bent at an acute angle, slightly elevated and about six to eight inches from your torso. It's recommended you then use your arms to shift your weight slightly as you run down the trail.

A SAMPLE VISUALIZATION PIECE FOR ATHLETES TO TRY

Most if not all sport psychology experts agree that mental training can enhance your running performance. Visualization is a key element with respect to mental preparation of races. It most certainly worked for me personally over the span of eight years prior to running a sub four-minute mile. Since the 10K distance is the more popular race distance for road runners, provided below is an example of how to use visualization to prepare for a 10k race.

Imagine yourself at the race site where you'll arrive wearing your sweats. Notice the sun, the clouds, and other runners. Feel yourself confident, relaxed, and looking forward to running your best, feeling fit and fast. You have been training hard and you are ready.

Imagine yourself warming up and doing your stretches and strides, lining up at the start. You hear the starter giving you instructions, noticing your opponents and feeling excited, exhilarated. Your muscles and body are ready to go. You feel the familiar excitement and take three deep breaths to calm yourself, as energy surges in your body. The gun sounds and you take off running for position. You take your time staying relaxed and fluid, but someone bumps your shoulder. You keep your form and balance, taking note of the other people around you.

Your stride is smooth, and you are centered, balanced and comfortable, enjoying the race and feeling powerful. You are practically floating and in complete control. Your mind is on your form and the runners around you. You hear your first mile split, and you are right on schedule. You glide along effortlessly feeling the uphills and the downhills. The miles progress along easily, two, three and you hear your time, you are doing well. You begin to push harder knowing this fourth mile is important, maintaining your form, your technique, and your breathing. You begin to surge, passing runners, finding yourself in better position and staying with the pack.

You pass the five-mile mark, hearing your time. You adjust according to your plan and strategy, your legs moving powerfully and your arms pumping up and down. You pick up your pace running hard and fast, knowing this is the crucial sixth mile in the race, keeping your focus and concentration, surging, passing and thanking your body for its strength . . . relaxing and striding long and powerful.

You pick it up again, the last half mile reaching down deep for your reserve into another gear, faster and faster until you are at the last quarter of a mile, and you begin to kick hard telling yourself what a great kick you have passing more people. You sprint through the finish line hearing the cheer of the crowd and feeling the exhilaration. You slow, catching your breath, your sides heaving. You jog slowly hearing congratulations from other runners and friends promising your body it will rest soon. YOU HAVE ACHIEVED YOUR GOAL!

MEDITATION TECHNIQUES TO SUPPORT YOUR RUNNING

Meditation quiets the mind, relaxes the body, and puts us in a non-judgmental, neutral but alert state. It's recommended the ultimate goal is to transcend the mind and discover the wisdom and tranquility within. Below are eight basic mediation steps:

1. Find a quiet environment free of distractions.

2. Sit in a comfortable position with your spine straight, your hands resting naturally on your lap.

3. Close eyes and focus each time you release a breath.

4. Slow down the breath, let any tension go with each exhalation.

5. Choose a word or phrase to recite slowly on each exhalation.

6. Notice distractions and acknowledge them as you let them pass and go back to your focus.

7. Begin with five minutes and work up to twenty to thirty minutes.

8. Have patience and remember there is no right or wrong way.

Being totally in focus and experiencing movements such as running as a moving meditation is also very beneficial so just relax and enjoy.

DETERMINING IF YOU SHOULD EXERCISE WHEN YOU ARE SICK

If you are a beginner or a competitive runner, knowing when to exercise if you don't feel well can be difficult. When you have an infection such as a cold or stomach flu you need to decide how exercise might affect your health and your road back to recovery. When your body is fighting an infection your performance and fitness benefits will likely be less than optimal. When this happens missing a few days of training is not the end of the world and the best option is not to run.

Sometimes physical activity can help you feel better. For example, running a short distance can sometimes temporarily clear head congestion when you have a cold. The times when you do think exercise might help, it's recommended you try the *"neck check"* for your symptoms. If your symptoms are located above the neck like a stuffy or runny nose, sneezing or a sore throat, then exercise is probably safe. It's recommended you start running conservatively and if you feel better after ten minutes then you can increase your pace and finish the workout. Obviously, if you feel really bad then stop running.

On the other hand, you may want to pay close attention to *"below the neck"* symptoms. It's recommended you avoid intense physical activity if you have muscle aches, hacking cough, chills, vomiting, diarrhea, and a fever of 100F or higher. Running when you have below the neck symptoms may result in feeling weak and dehydrated. It's recommended that athletes can resume running when below the neck symptoms subside; however, when recovering from an illness that prevented you from running, it's important to ease back into activity gradually. A good rule to follow is to exercise for two days at a lower-than-normal intensity for each day you are sick. From my personal experience when feeling the cold and flu type symptoms both of these "neck check" approaches have worked remarkably well when executed over the years.

ACCLIMATING TO RUNNING IN HOT WEATHER

Various studies have shown that if you do not live in a hot and humid climate you will be at a significant disadvantage when you race in that environment unless you acclimate. Heat acclimatization will allow increased work output by reducing your core body temperature during the race, increasing your sweat production, beginning sweat production earlier, helping your body conserve salt, and conserving muscle glycogen. It takes seven to fourteen days to completely acclimate with fitter people leaning toward the shorter time. You don't need to train in heat every day, but don't go more than two to three days between heat sessions. The type of exercise is not important, but sessions lasting at least sixty minutes, with about 100 minutes being optimal, is important. Shorten the intensity and duration of your workouts for at least the first three to five days of acclimatization. Reduce your warm-up intensity and duration for the entire process to prevent your core temperature from rising too high before training or racing.

A question often asked is what if you live in a cooler climate and cannot take two weeks off work? Your normal training will help. Regularly raising your core temperature by hitting an intensity over 50 percent of your VO2 max with strenuous interval training or continuous exercise will invoke heat acclimatization responses, but eight to twelve weeks are needed to really do the job. Remember your need for fluid will still increase despite acclimatization, and electrolyte or sports drinks have been proven to be more effective due to preferred taste in keeping you hydrated and moving than plain water. Drink both water and sports drinks throughout the days leading up to the race and be sure to stay hydrated during the race itself.

SLEEPING BENEFITS FOR IMPROVED RUNNING PERFORMANCE

Brian Owen was quoted as saying, "Training is what you are doing while your opponent is sleeping in," and this quote has been shared many times amongst many runners and coaches over the years. However, sufficient adequate sleep is critically important toward the success of every athlete's performance. Each of us has slightly different sleep requirements. Some do fine on four hours and a short nap, but seven to eight hours is sufficient for most of us. More than eight hours of sleep at one time not only makes us sluggish but can be a waste of valuable time. Recent research has found that short naps of one hour or less are very beneficial in improving alertness and mood for the remainder of the day. If you wake at 6:00 a.m., around 3:00 p.m. is the ideal time for a nap, so it's recommended you experiment and see what works best for you.

The ideal sleeping position is on your side with head resting on a pillow in line with your spine. Top leg bent and bottom leg slightly flexed. On your back is the second-best position. Try to never sleep of your stomach; it compresses the spine and restricts breathing. Stretching and relaxing while thinking positive thoughts before bed is an excellent way to prepare for a healing and restful sleep. In benefiting from adequate sleep, you will be able to train and race more effectively.

TRAINING HARDER IS NOT ALWAYS BETTER

Many ambitious runners might share with you that workouts are good when you run the intervals faster, reducing the rest interval or both. This method will make the workout harder, but it will also make it less effective. If you want to train your anaerobic system, then your faster workout with shorter recovery is the way to go because you will be running much of your workout anaerobically. If your goal is to improve your aerobic system, the one that is primarily focused on your target races of 5K to 10K then your hard work on the track is partially a loss. The reason being is that you are not providing the boost to your V02 max that you could be, therefore you are limiting your ability to reach your potential in races.

You may wonder why you consistently race slower than your workout times would predict while a friend who is slower in workouts but is actually training at his V02 max pace beats them when it counts in races. This is possible because if you work overly hard on the track in the middle of the week, it will likely leave you too tired to recover in time for weekend races, while your friend who does workouts at the hard but proper pace can absorb the benefits of training and recover enough in a few days to race well on the weekend.

CROSS-TRAINING ADVANTAGES

My one personal regret during the 1980s and '90s while participating in track and field is that I did not engage enough in cross-training type activities. Furthermore, I suspect many competitive high school and college runners after the first running boom in the 1970s chose to run every day of the week, rather than incorporate a cross-training activity like swimming or cycling into their training regimen.

It definitely was not part of my own vocabulary throughout high school or college. I believe this has changed and running experts including myself now realize that cross-training offers tremendous advantages for both competitive athletes and those who train simply to keep in shape and manage their weight. Cross-training helps you to do the following:

1. Add variety to workouts to maintain interest.

2. Use traditional training methods like running and swimming along with exercising using various machines.

3. Develop the entire body, rather than specific parts of energy systems (aerobic vs anaerobic).

4. Distribute the load of training among various body parts thus reducing the risk of injury.

5. Keep training while injured. When one body part is injured, runners can train using different muscles and joints.

6. Train indoors if the weather is inappropriate. There are no excuses.

CROSS TRAINING AND TOTAL BODY CONDITIONING THROUGH STRENGTH TRAINING BENEFITS

The related benefits of cross-training and total body conditioning through strength training are important elements to realize. Below are the key benefits:

1. **Increase in muscle mass:** The increase in lean muscle mass that results from strength training is the key to the body's ability to metabolize glucose and thus burn fat. This occurs because muscle cells require more energy than fat cells.

2. **Body composition changes:** Muscular strength declines approximately 5 percent per decade for the untrained individual. Strength training slows down this process, even as people reach their senior years.

3. **Bone protection:** Weight training helps protect bones. This is an important benefit, particularly for women as decreased estrogen production causes bone demineralization. This in turn increases the risks of osteoporosis and the additional risk of incurring stress fractures. Muscles that impact on bone structure as a result of weight training facilitates bone regeneration.

4. **Diabetes and heart disease prevention:** According to the literature, weight training seems to reduce the risk factors for adult-onset diabetes and heart disease.

Reference: *Everyday Health Newsletter. "Strength Training Found to Lower Heart Disease and Diabetes Risk, Whether or Not You Do Cardio" by Don Rauf, March 25, 2019.*

RESEARCH SUPPORTS THE BENEFITS OF CROSS-TRAINING

Although cross-training seems to make perfect sense, not all experts agree on its benefits. Cross-training contradicts the time-honored principle that training should be limited in scope and closely aligned to the performance your clients want to improve. In other words, if athletes want to be good distance runners, they need to run mainly long distances.

According to this principle, non-specific activities for runners like weight training or swimming are wasted effort because they do not make someone a better runner. Obviously, most coaches including myself disagree with this thought process and recent research demonstrates that a well-balanced program will enhance your primary activity. Besides, the typical fitness enthusiast is interested in total body conditioning rather than sport specific training.

Many sports scientists believe that cross-training may lead to optimal effort because peak performance in any physical activity usually involves more than one physical attribute. For example, a marathoner may need a strong sprint to the finish line which requires high levels of aerobic and anaerobic fitness. Furthermore, weight training can help reduce upper body muscle fatigue while running. A strong upper body helps minimize fatigue and stiffness in the arms, shoulders, and neck areas and that, in turn, enables a runner to maintain form late in a marathon or long run. Legs move only as fast as the arms swing.

The runner with a strong upper body will find more power for the sprint to the finish line, an easier effort uphill, and better balance when running on trails. You'll be surprised how far you can go from the point where you thought it ended. All of these add up to an ability to run faster and more efficiently.

CROSS-TRAINING BENEFITS RUNNERS

Exercise can provide a total body tune-up. It can strengthen the heart, bones, muscles, and joints. It can enhance cardiovascular fitness, build muscle, reduce body fat, and improve flexibility. Many experts would agree that cross-training is critical if these gains are to be met. In cross-training, two or more types of exercise are performed in one workout or used alternatively in successive workouts. A distance runner in training may also lift weights twice a week, perform daily stretching exercises, and perform high intensity bicycle sprints once a week.

Runners also turn to cross-training to fight boredom but also because no single exercise can yield all the potential benefits of many runners. For example, with respect to running it certainly enhances aerobic fitness, which in turn improves cardiovascular health and requires sustained use of large muscle groups like those in the legs. What's interesting is that running contributes little to developing muscle mass, especially in the upper body.

Running also creates a slight muscular imbalance in the legs, as the hamstrings and calf muscles develop at a faster rate than the quadriceps and shins. Weight training helps address this imbalance. Additionally, strong quadriceps and hips help protect these areas from a variety of injuries that include IT band syndrome; strong legs also offer protection from the possibility of injury when running at a fast pace downhill.

THE BENEFITS OF WATER RUNNING

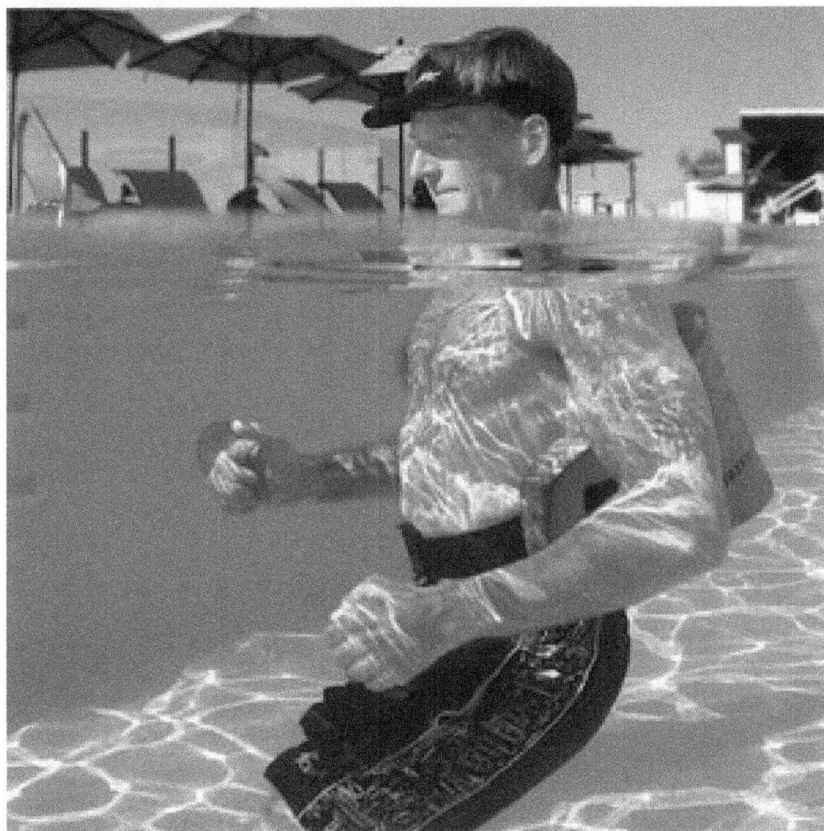

Aqua jogging is the closest simulated activity to actual running on surfaces that you can find. Use water jogging as cross-training to supplement your road running, or use it as a running replacement, if injured.

What is aqua jogging? Aqua jogging, aka deep water running, is a form of cardiovascular exercise that mimics the motion of jogging while submerged in water. You can do aqua jogging by running laps in the pool or wearing a flotation device around your trunk and running in place. Leading up to the

1992 US Olympic Trials, I strained my calf muscle, subsequently preventing me from doing intervals or any kind of speed work. While recovering from the calf injury I spent every day in the pool doing water running workouts and this maintained the fitness I needed to be competitive at the Olympic Trials that year. What makes aqua jogging so effective is that it allows you to "run" without landing on a hard surface. For example, if you have an injury such as Achilles' tendonitis, knee soreness, and ankle sprains, etc., then water jogging provides you with the ability to engage in running movement without the pounding, allowing your body to heal.

Two key recommendations for water running are: (1) Use a flotation device such as an aqua jog belt to maintain proper running form. Without something to hold you upright, you risk compromising your form and developing bad habits. (2) Wear a heart rate monitor so that you can easily gauge your effort level. Due to buoyancy, your heart rate in the water is about ten to fifteen beats per minute lower than it would be on land for the same effort.

BELOW IS AN EXAMPLE OF A WORKOUT YOU CAN DO IN THE POOL

Fartlek interval workout = ten-minute warmup, then a set of 10x1-minute hard intervals with thirty seconds rest between each hard minute. Then proceed with another set of 5x2-minute hard intervals with thirty seconds in between. The last set is of 3x3-minute hard intervals with thirty seconds in between. End with a ten-minute cool down.

Bonus recommendations are to find a pool where there is some music or find a training partner to join you. Workouts in the water can be a fun alternative to the road. When finished, you can recover knowing you did effective work in the pool and will see positive long-term fitness results.

PRECAUTIONS AND CONSIDERATIONS FOR CROSS-TRAINING

Runners should start slowly with single activities that are varied and this will allow a progression to cross-training without causing injury or undue fatigue. As a runner you need to be sure you do not have any past or underlying injuries that would cause problems by cross-training. The worst-case scenario is to worsen a condition or delay the healing process if you happen to be injured.

Some cross-training options when incorporated carefully into a runner's workout routine will enhance overall training. Remember, it's vital that runners receive instruction on the correct use of equipment. Furthermore, to receive the maximum benefit while minimizing chances of incurring injury, it is also important that runners perform activities using proper form, technique, and posture.

THE BENEFITS OF CYCLING, SWIMMING, ELLIPTIGO AND AQUA JOGGING

The following activities are great cross-training options that when included into your routine will enhance overall training. Below are the cross-training benefits for cycling, swimming, ElliptiGO and aqua jogging.

Cycling involves running related muscle groups such as the quadriceps and shins, both of which don't develop as rapidly as the calf muscles and hamstrings. Cycling also strengthens the connective tissue of the knee, hip, and ankle regions, thus, reducing the risk of injury. Cycling will also build great strength in the glutes without producing the same high impact forces as running, but it still challenges the cardiovascular system extensively. After a stressful run, cycling also loosens fatigued leg muscles. Since it's much more difficult to run after cycling, run first before getting on a bike. Cycling helps runners avoid those common injuries that tend to occur with the higher running volumes necessary for great racing performance. After my track racing career was over, I cycled over both the Swiss and Italian Alps in 2006 and 2008.

Swimming is one of the best cross-training activities, for several reasons. Swimming enables exercisers to build muscular strength and endurance while improving flexibility. It's recommended that athletes who want to prevent injury or are pregnant or are recovering from an injury, suffering from joint or bone conditions or are overweight should exercise in a weightless environment. Swimming reduces the effects of poor posture because it's necessary to stretch out from head to toes in order to glide through the water. Keep in mind that, compared to other cross-training activities, runners' heart rates may not reach as high a level while swimming due to the loss of gravitational force, the horizontal position, and the cooling effect of the water temperature. Swimming is often a good choice when recovering from an injury.

ElliptiGO bike is a weight-bearing, low-impact cross-training tool that closely simulates the running motion and provides a highly efficient workout. It complements the same muscular contractions as running in a way no other cross-training device can. The pedaling motion distributes force evenly through the feet and engages more of the hamstrings and glutes than traditional cycling. A ride on an ElliptiGO bike is a full-body workout that burns 33 percent more calories than riding a traditional bike, without the back, neck and seat pain commonly associated with cycling. In fact, many describe the experience as "running on air." Runners can train longer and harder on an ElliptiGO bike with a lower risk of injuries. ElliptiGO bikes can be ridden outdoors, or indoors with the addition of a stationary trainer. Experience the joy of running without the negative effects of impact. *Contributing Author for the above excerpt is Bryce Whiting, Chief Enthusiast at ElliptioGO Inc.*

Aqua jogging is perfect for rehabilitating many injuries due to the fact there is no shock from foot strike, and water running is a great alternative to dryland running activities. Aqua jogging promotes extensive cardiovascular benefits without stressing the legs very much at all. Due to the fact the movement replicates running very closely, your cardiovascular gains have a much better transfer to running. It's also good for your psyche because it closely approximates the running movement. For either purpose, it should be based on the runner's current level of ability. Aqua jog belts are definitely recommended thus making the workout easier.

THE BASIC AEROBIC WORKOUT USING THE STATIONARY BIKE

During my sophomore year in college, I pulled my calf muscle while competing in the 800 meters at the University of Southern California. Although I was not able to run for the next six weeks, I did continue to exercise using the stationary bike. My recommendation is to begin by adjusting the seat height, so the leg has a slight bend on the knee when the foot touches the pedal at its lowest point. The leg should extend as much as possible, without locking the knee. Hips should not rock from side to side to extend leg. Begin pedaling, keeping shoulders relaxed and knees in line with your feet.

It's recommended you warm-up for two minutes at low tension and rpms to prepare the body. Gradually increase the speed and if needed the tension and the emphasis is on speed. The tension should be as light as needed to achieve target heart rate while maintaining a minimum 80 rpm. The key is to find the speed and tension combination that can be maintained at your target heart rate and after three minutes of the program your pulse should be taken. Pulse rate should be increasing, but you should never be out of breath for any length of time.

It's estimated that after approximately four more minutes you should be at or close to your target heart rate. Find your pulse rate, adjusting tension and speed accordingly and maintain this rate for the duration, determined by fitness level and cardiovascular endurance. This duration should gradually increase, one minute each workout up to thirty to sixty minutes, depending on heart rate recovery.

USING THE STATIONARY BIKE IMPROVES YOUR FITNESS

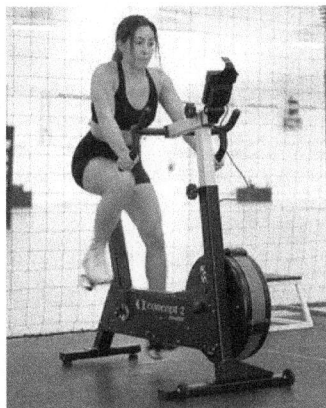

Research shows that cycling workouts can boost max V02 by up to 15 percent and cut your 5K and 10K times by as much as 9 percent. Below are two great workouts to improve race times:

Workout #1: This one's for the legs. Warm-up with ten minutes of easy pedaling and then stand up and pedal at close to maximum intensity against tough resistance for 1 minute. Recover with two minutes of easy pedaling, then repeat. Start with four work intervals and eventually work up to ten. Cool down with ten minutes of easy cycling.

Workout #2: This one's for your heart. Warm-up for ten minutes, then pedal continuously for twenty to thirty minutes at 85 percent of your maximum heart rate while cycling. Since your max heart rate while running is normally about ten beats higher than your maximum heart rate while cycling, you'll actually be at about 90 percent of maximum cycling heart rate. As you progress, increase to forty minutes of hard pedaling and always remember to warm-down.

After six weeks of no running due to my calf injury in college at USC, I was able to run a 4:17 mile and this happened after exercising solely on the stationary bike. Exercising on the stationary bike definitely maintains one's fitness.

THE STAIR CLIMBER HAS ADDED FITNESS BENEFITS

In some recent studies, subjects who did only stair climbing workouts for nine weeks improved running performance as much as a second group who did running workouts. Below are two great stair climbing workouts:

Workout #1: To bolster leg muscle power, warm-up with ten minutes of easy jogging on the treadmill. Stretch lightly for two minutes and focus on your quadriceps, jog again for a minute or two, then climb aboard the stair climber. Give yourself a minute to get comfortable, then go hard for two minutes at a hard 5K effort feeling. Recover with easy climbing for two minutes, then go hard again. Try for four work intervals the first session, eventually working up to ten.

Workout #2: To increase leg muscle endurance, warm up as indicated above, then climb for twenty to twenty-five minutes at about 85 percent of maximum heart rate. After a month or two, you should be able to do thirty-five to forty minutes.

For both of these workouts simply cool down by walking on the treadmill or your outside environment. After doing these workouts you'll have done less pounding on the roads and your legs will be better rested too.

ADDITIONAL CROSS-TRAINING BENEFITS OF ROWING, STAIRMASTER, VERSA CLIMBER, ELLIPTICAL AND WALKING

As discussed, there are other great cross-training options that when included into your routine will enhance overall training. Below are the cross-training benefits for the rowing machine, stair-master, versa climber, elliptical trainer, and walking.

Rowing machine: Rowing is another great cardiovascular activity. It strengthens the hips, buttocks, and upper body, while sparing the legs of heavy pounding. Be sure to learn proper rowing technique to maximize the benefits of this activity.

Stairmaster: Stairmaster provides a great cardiovascular workout while being rather gentle on the skeletal system. To achieve maximum benefits, proper form and posture must be used. For an even more intense and regulated step, you can try the step mill machine.

Versa Climber: Using a versa climber provided a total body workout because all the major muscles of the upper and lower body are fully engaged and thus strengthened. Because of this coordination required by the arms and legs it can be a challenging machine to learn to use correctly. Be sure to learn proper technique.

Elliptical Trainer: Elliptical trainers provide a great total body cardiovascular workout. Their oval like motion provides the runner with the feel of classic cross-country skiing, stairclimbing, and walking — all in combination. The elliptical trainer can be programmed to operate in either a forward or backward motion, providing a low impact workout for all the major muscles in the legs. The backward motion emphasizes the gluteal muscles (buttocks). Athletes can achieve a great upper body workout by using the two poles located on each side of the machine in conjunction with the leg motion.

Walking: Walking provides great therapeutic benefits following a hard workout or a rest day. Walking is also a great way to initiate clients to a training program. It builds confidence while decreasing apprehension to exercise and fatigue the following day. Walking is the most popular form of exercise and for most people it's safe, easy to stay consistent with, and has very minimal costs.

USING THE TREADMILL FOR AN AEROBIC WORKOUT

As a runner there are times when you want to break from the hard pavement and it's at these times you can get quality work through two challenging workouts that is recommended below for you to try on the treadmill. It's important to create your own variations and do one per week and rest assured you'll be more than ready for your next competition.

The treadmill enables you to run indoors and with considerably less pounding than on the roads. Here I am providing two workouts for you to consider doing in the future.

Workout #1: For a great power workout first warm-up for ten minutes then set the treadmill at twenty to twenty-five seconds per mile slower than your usual 10K race pace. Run for three minutes with the incline at zero and switch the incline to 2 percent and run for one minute. Switch to 4 percent and go for another minute. Go to 6 percent for a final minute, then return to the flat for three minutes. Try to do these sets of 2-4-6 for your first session, eventually working up to seven or eight sets.

Workout #2: This workout is great for endurance. Warm up for five to ten minutes, then do a mile at your most recent 10K race pace with the incline set at 1 percent. Recover with four minutes of easy jogging, then repeat the mile two more times. As your endurance improves, shorten the recoveries to two or three minutes or nudge up the incline to 2 or 3 percent.

HOW DO I BEST GAIN WEIGHT?

There are a few times during my teaching and coaching career when students and athletes alike personally inquire about how to gain weight. To gain weight, you have to consistently eat more calories than when you are maintaining weight. The easiest way to do this is to drink extra fluids like low-fat milk or juices. Cranberry juice is particularly high in calories. Furthermore, the carbohydrates in juices provide lots of energy for muscle building exercise that helps you gain weight.

You can also eat extra snacks and larger portions of meals. You don't need expensive weight gain drinks, they are simply high-priced calories in a can. It's recommended you simply eat and drink 500 to 1000 more calories per day of wholesome foods.

IS IT POSSIBLE FOR SLOW-TWITCH FIBERS TO BE CONVERTED INTO FAST-TWITCH FIBERS?

In 1991, I was fortunate to qualify for the National British 1500-meter AAA Championships that took place in Birmingham, England. I took great pride in qualifying for this event since my father would watch these same championships as a kid . . . and now he got to watch his own son. I felt so honored as I lined up in lane one next to the reigning world record holder in the men's mile, Steve Cram in lane two. As I toed the line in that championship race, I reflected back to ten years earlier in 1981 at Saint Augustine High School on my first day of practice as a ninth grader and recognized back then and now to present day that I was blessed with fast twitch fibers where I'm racing against the best athletes in the world. I ended up finishing just a couple seconds behind Steve Cram that day. It was a thrill of a lifetime!

The notion that one type of muscle fiber can be converted into another type of fiber is the subject of considerable debate. On the one hand coaches who are in favor or performing fast speed movements believe for example that lifting weights explosively will convert slow twitch fibers into fast twitch fibers. There is no scientific evidence that consistently supports this notion that slow twitch fibers or vice versa.

It appears as if one type of muscle fiber may take on certain metabolic characteristics of another type of muscle fiber, but an actual conversion does not occur. In other words, you cannot convert one fiber type into another any more than you can convert a donkey into a gazelle. If you were to take a donkey and train it like a cheetah, you might get a slightly faster donkey, but you will never get a cheetah.

HOW MUCH SHOULD YOU WEIGH & THE BEST EXERCISE FOR WEIGHT LOSS

Due to the fact weight is largely under genetic control, look at your immediate and extended family. Genetics aside, the rule of thumb to estimate appropriate weight is as follows:

Women: 100 pounds for the first five feet of height plus five pounds for every inch thereafter.

Men: 106 pounds for the first five feet of height plus six pounds for every inch thereafter.

This means a 5'8 women should weigh around 140 pounds, and a 5'8 man, 154 pounds. This formula, though, does not account for bone structure and musculature. Furthermore, add or subtract 10 percent if you have a large or small bone or muscle structure.

Is running the best exercise for weight loss? Is it walking or aerobics? The best exercise for weight loss is one you enjoy doing. To lose weight, burn more calories than you engage on a regular basis. The more you like a physical activity, the more likely you will stay with it.

INCREASING YOUR METABOLISM THROUGH EXERCISE

Body composition is a question of energy balance, which means calories consumed must equal calories burned to maintain weight. The rate of expenditure of energy can vary from person to person. We expend energy not only during exercise but during every second of our lives. These seconds add up to years just as a few extra calories a day can add up to several extra pounds of body fat. For this reason, metabolic rate is an important factor in the energy balance equation.

By definition, metabolic rate is how fast your body uses and produces energy which is the rate it burns calories. Metabolic rate is highest during intense exercise and lowest when you are sleeping. It varies with size, age, heredity, body composition, activity level, food intake and weight loss history. During exercise, metabolic rate can be more than ten times higher than resting levels. Thirty minutes of vigorous exercise can burn the same number of calories as five hours of sitting at your desk. For example, extra calories are burned when you climb a flight of stairs instead of taking the elevator and small amounts of exercise can add up to a significant effect on metabolic rate throughout the day. Metabolic rate may also remain elevated for several hours if you have worked out consistently at 60 to 80 percent of aerobic capacity for more than thirty to forty minutes.

One of the best things exercise can do is increase the amount of muscle you have and since muscle is metabolically more active than fat, the greater your lean body mass, the higher your metabolic rate. Exercise greatly enhances weight loss efforts because of its tremendous physiological and psychological benefits; therefore, exercise helps burn fat. It decreases appetite and makes you feel more energetic and look better. Decrease in metabolic rate that occurs with age is due to a decrease in activity and a loss of muscle from lack of exercise. Simply stated metabolic rate slows down in people who slow down. After running my last mile on May 31, 2022, and undergoing a hip replacement, my biggest challenge was identifying an activity other than running that met the same exercise activity levels I was used to for forty-two years. Walking three to four miles every day is now a great alternative exercise for me and it's easy on the joints. During this stage of life my fitness goals are now centered toward the emphasis of health promotion rather than on the importance of exercise achievement. It's important to continue exercising for its long-term effects on metabolism and health.

VARIETY OF EXERCISE IS CRITICAL FOR SUCCESS

To enjoy running to its fullest, which is necessary if you wish to make a lifelong fitness commitment, your training routes must provide variety. For variety purposes, it doesn't mean that every run has to be different. We all develop certain familiar routes that we repeat many times. Your running needs to contain an element of exploration so from time to time you should venture into different parks, beaches, new neighborhoods, and other areas off the beaten path.

These places are likely to include a few hills, so run them. Running on the flat ground all the time can be boring so moderate hill running will add spice to your training. When you travel to another city it's recommended to run to the top of the nearest big hill while running easily up it and enjoying all the surroundings, and as you reach the top you are rewarded with hopefully a scenic view. Daily exercise delivers endless rewards. That said, we are all human and may sometimes get bored in our workout routine. Your typical running routes may become burdensome and monotonous. When I experience these feelings of dread, I escape to the beach in Del Mar and run during the sunrise or sunset where the peaceful hum of the ocean waves centers my soul. These are special moments that invigorate my love of fitness and fill me with gratitude to be alive and healthy. The greatest form of prayer is gratitude.

EXERCISING IN SUBFREEZING AIR

During the wintertime in many parts of the United States, people enjoy heading to the mountains to ski. For athletes, skiing may not be enough, and you might want to exercise in subfreezing air. The question arises of whether it is dangerous to exercise in subfreezing air. In short, it can be dangerous to exercise in subfreezing air and if you're prone to exercise-induced asthma or angina, cold air can precipitate an attack. A light scarf or ski mask pulled loosely in front of your mouth can help warm up air. Another danger is dehydration, which will hinder the body's ability to regulate its temperature. When you're active, you lose fluids by sweating and particularly in winter by breathing.

The dry winter air has to be warmed and moistened by the respiratory system. As you exhale you lose water and when you can see your breath, you're seeing water droplets. Furthermore, urine production is stimulated by the cold. It's recommended you drink plenty of nonalcoholic beverages when exercising.

RECOMMENDED FREQUENCY AND TIME FOR EXERCISE

Most studies show that exercising thirty minutes on most days each week is what it takes to improve fitness; however, sometimes it's easier to make exercise a habit if you do it every day.

With exercise, harder is not better, but longer workouts are recommended so if you want fast improvement, exercise longer rather than harder. Although you can get good fitness benefits from as little as ten minutes of exercise per day, extending your exercise time will increase your rewards. This is especially true for up to one hour of exercise per day. Beyond that, there may be diminishing health returns and increasing risk of injuries.

Another approach to exercise is to remain active and make active choices when there are options. For example, walk upstairs as opposed to using the elevator or walk from the back of a parking lot at your local grocery store instead of trying to park right in front of the store. This makes a difference too.

"The ultimate measure of a person is not where they stand in moments of comfort and convenience, but where they stand at times of challenge and controversy."

— Dr. Martin Luther King

TIPS ON TRAINING
FOR A RACE

5K WORKOUT HELPS IMPROVE RACE PERFORMANCE

Oprah Winfrey was once quoted as saying, *"Running is the greatest metaphor for life, because you get out of it what you put into it."* If you want to improve your 5K time, then I recommend this great workout for runners. Find a large open, grassy area and you will need to measure and mark a loop approximately 1000 meters long. After a thorough warm-up my recommendation is to run the first loop at your current personal 5K race pace and then jog easily for five minutes. Run the second 1000-meter loop about three seconds faster.

Continue in this manner by dropping down by three seconds each loop with five minutes' rest between loops. I recommend aiming for five loops total. Make sure you warm down after this difficult workout. Furthermore, be sure to mark a point about halfway around the loop where you can check you are on pace. This workout is great for beginning runners because it teaches them to run at 5K pace or faster. Tuesdays are the best day to run this workout before a weekend race since this leaves you more time to recover.

A 10K WORKOUT THAT HELPS IMPROVE RACE PERFORMANCE

This workout is difficult, but it's perfectly adaptable for anyone hoping to improve in the 10K distance and the workout below was beneficial that led me to run a 29:30 personal best for the 10K. Below is a 10K workout that will work for you:

Over a measured 10-kilometer stretch, alternate two-minute surges at your current 10K race pace with one-minute jog rest intervals. At the end of the 10K I recommend you warm down for ten minutes.

This workout works great because running at 10K pace for about 70 percent of the 10K distance increases max Vo2 boosts running efficiency and improves neuromuscular coordination, yet you will not feel wasted afterward. Perhaps most importantly, zipping through most of a 10K at race pace intensity will really increase your confidence.

I recommend you try this workout once a week during the month before your racing season begins.

400 REPEATS LEAD TO FASTER 5K PERFORMANCES

It's definitely true that 5K type workouts develop stamina, increased speed, and a sense of pace. Another potential workout you can do once a week is to select a track or separately measured stretch of path or road.

I recommend jogging easily for ten minutes, then do 400-meter repeats at one to three seconds per lap faster than your current 5K pace. When running this pace, it's not what you want to run but what you can run. After each repeat, recover with an easy 400-meter jog.

When you finish the 400s be sure to cool down with a mile or longer of easy running. Begin with four to six 400s and add one every two weeks until you reach ten or twelve. A variation at that point would be to reduce the rest interval to 300 meters, drop the number of repeats back down to six, and begin climbing again.

My experience in prescribing 400 repeats is that most runners enjoy the distance of this interval and gain great fitness benefits completing them.

INCREASED POWER TRANSLATES TO FASTER RACING PERFORMANCES & BENEFITS OF INTERVAL CUT DOWNS

Improved power translates to a quicker foot strike and longer strides. One learns that reducing foot strike time by two hundredths of a second and increasing stride length by a half inch will reduce fifteen minutes from a mudpack marathoner's race time.

The most effective way to increase your power is with hill work and preferably once a week. I recommend on your hill running days, combine high-speed approaches up steep hills with more moderate, continuous running on less steep hills. You might want to consider adding some plyometric drills too. Uphill bounding along with exaggerated hopping and high knee skipping are all effective plyometric drills.

Recent research suggests that runners who build up high levels of lactate early in a race tend to run their 8K or 10K races about 2.5 percent slower than usual. The question remains how do you learn leg turnover rate and the feeling of effort associated with your goal race pace?

It's my belief running 800-meter repeats at your goal race pace, while concentrating on how the pace feels, is effective and beneficial. After each 800, check your watch to see if you have been running faster or slower than race pace. By adjusting your speed on subsequent repeats, you will eventually lock into the proper pace and develop a better feel for it.

Furthermore, I recommend running "cut downs" to gain experience with race pace. To do these, run 1200 repeats, first starting at slower than race pace and gradually increasing the speed on each successive repeat until you are running slightly faster than race pace. You can avoid burnout by running no more than four to six miles per week of these repeats.

OVERCOMING YOUR RACE PACE PROBLEMS

Once you become accustomed to your race pace in workouts, one difficult problem remains. The pace almost feels easier in a race than it does in a workout. For this reason, I recommend it's often best to run a little slower than you think you should during the first mile of a race. Keep in mind the pace may feel sluggish, but chances are that it feels slow because of the excitement of the race and that in reality it's very close to the pace you're aiming for in the race.

My recommendation on race day is to settle into your goal pace and run steadily through the opening two miles. Once you have familiarized yourself with race pace, your confidence will grow, your performances will become more consistent, and your race times will improve.

I learned this most when training and racing with my Saint Augustine high school and San Diego State University teammates and training every day with Steve Scott — who has run more sub four-minute miles than anyone in history.

Reference: Runners Tribe. *137 Sub-4 Minute Milers the Training of Steve Scott.* By Runnerstribe Admin. April 1, 2018.

THE IMPORTANCE OF ACCLIMATING TO HEAT BEFORE RACING

American track and field coach and co-founder of Nike, Bill Bowerman, once said, *"There is no such thing as bad weather, just soft people."* Various studies have shown that if you do not live in a hot and humid climate you will be more at a significant disadvantage when you race in that environment, unless you acclimate. Heat acclimatization will allow increased work output by reducing your core body temperature during the race, increasing your sweat production, beginning sweat production earlier, helping your body conserve salt, and conserving muscle glycogen.

It takes seven to fourteen days to completely acclimate, with fitter people leaning towards the shorter time. You don't need to train in hot weather every day, but don't go more than two to three days between heat sessions. The type of exercise is not important but sessions lasting at least sixty minutes with about 100 minutes being optimal is important. I recommend shortening the intensity and duration of your workout for at least the first three to five days of acclimatization. Reduce your warm-up intensity and duration for the entire process to prevent your core temperature from rising too high before training or racing.

The 1992 US Olympic Track and Field Trials were held in New Orleans and took place in late June, when it's hot. In leading up to the 1500-meter event at those trials, I completed all of my running workouts midday during the hottest time in San Diego.

THE MARATHON EFFECTS ON THE IMMUNE SYSTEM

Microscopic damage to the muscles from running a marathon can cause more than soreness. The muscle damage incurred from running a marathon can divert some immune cells for muscle repair and weaken others, leaving the immune system less able to protect against upper respiratory tract infections.

While there is no direct evidence that those runners with the most weakened immune system are those who develop upper respiratory tract infections, there is evidence of a higher rate of it in marathon runners compared with non-runners. There is research suggesting that running a marathon depletes the immune system for three to seventy-two hours and thus increases the susceptibility to upper respiratory tract infections. Free radicals, byproducts of aerobic metabolism, also appear to play a role in promoting the muscle-damage induced inflammatory response. There is evidence that antioxidants like vitamin C combat free radicals and may help prevent a post marathon weakening of the immune system.

Running a marathon temporarily suppresses the immune system, but is the suppression great enough to increase the risk for developing upper respiratory tract infections? Below are guidelines for marathon runners that will improve and maintain your immune system.

1. Keep other life stresses to a minimum.

2. Eat a well-balanced diet.

3. Obtain adequate sleep.

4. Avoid putting hands to eyes and nose.

5. Avoid sick people and large crowds.

6. Avoid overtraining and rapid weight loss.

7. Use carbohydrate beverages before, during, and after marathon races and long training runs.

8. Wash your hands frequently.

TIPS AND TECHNIQUES THAT YOU NEED TO HAVE YOUR BEST RACE EVER

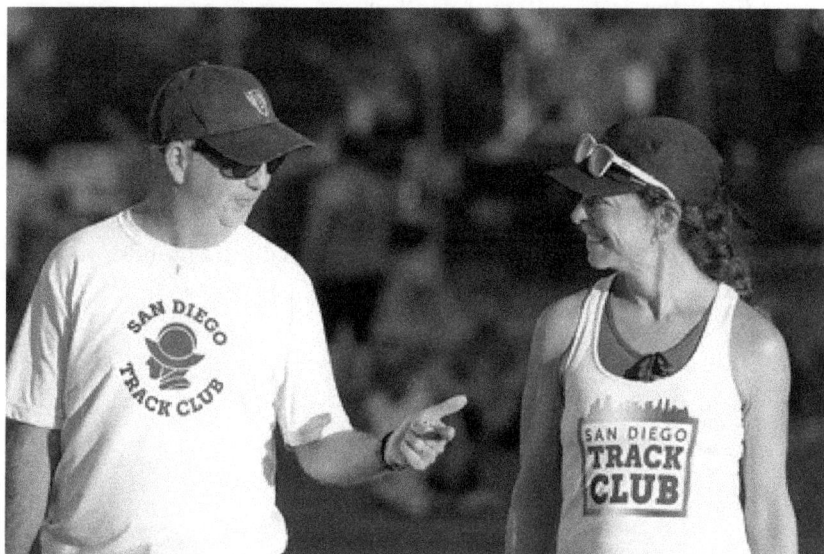

Over the past twenty-five years I have coached an estimated 15,000 marathoners so provided below are ten last-minute tips that you need to have your best race ever.

1. Running a marathon is all about energy conservation.

2. Drive the course to familiarize the route.

3. Do not skip any meals but do not overeat either.

4. Arrive at the start early.

5. You can determine if you are drinking enough water by monitoring your urine and it should be like clear lemonade.

6. Run in the middle of the road during your race.

7. Relax shoulders.

8. Try not to get discouraged when your race gets tough. Just know that discomfort is part of what you feel in a marathon, and you are not alone.

9. Do not panic at the start if your perceived pace is too slow. Conserve your energy and run with the flow of the pack for the first few miles.

10. Finally, the marathon is like a victory lap. The real rewards come from the training and accomplishments, milestones, and friends you make throughout your journeys.

PREPARING FOR THE LONGEST AND MOST IMPORTANT RUN OF THE YEAR

Three or four weeks before you race the marathon should mark the longest training run up to the 26.2-mile event. The long run is the most important day in any marathon-training program. In fact, more than any other workout, this is the one that prepares you for the physical and mental challenges of the marathon distance. In June 2007 I completed my first and only marathon and the twenty-mile run that I did four weeks before that marathon instilled in me tremendous confidence.

Long runs should make up 20 to 30 percent of your total weekly workouts, so for that weekend, provided you are prepared and ready, the recommended distance for this run is twenty-two miles. You should run far enough to prepare yourself for the marathon, but not so far that you become injured or over trained. It's recommended beginning marathoners run no more than three and a half hours, intermediate runners no more than three hours, and advanced runners no more than two and half hours during a training cycle.

If you're a beginner marathoner, you should do the longest run of the training program at a pace thirty to sixty seconds per mile slower than your current 10K race pace. If you're an intermediate or advanced marathoner, you should run at least sixty to ninety seconds slower than your 10K pace. Below are eight helpful tips on preparing for the longest run of the year:

1. No hard activity the night before this run. It's recommended you stay home and relax.

2. Treat this run like the race itself and plan to wear the same clothing and equipment that you will wear at your projected marathon.

3. Make sure you eat food or drink about one and half hours before the start of the run. That way you won't have a heavy feeling in your stomach.

4. Run on flat terrain this long run weekend and if possible, avoid hills.

5. Regarding water intake, it's recommended you drink a half to full liter per hour, which warrants 300 milligrams up to a gram of salt for optimal uptake and muscle hydration.

6. After one to two hours of running, carbohydrates should be definitely consumed.

7. Upon completion of the run stretch immediately. Hold the static stretches for a minimum of twenty to thirty seconds.

8. For food replenishment after the long run consume low-fat chocolate milk or a thick smoothie.

FINAL WEEK'S MARATHON PREPARATION

Below are a few pre-marathon tips that hopefully lead to a safe and successful race. During the week of the marathon and prior to the 26.2-mile race itself, you should consider this your week to rest, gradually decreasing your mileage so that by race day, your legs and body are well rested. While many runners are worried about weight gain during tapering, this is no time to be cutting back on meals. Choose from lean meats such as chicken and fish and high carbohydrate foods like rice, bagels, potatoes, and pancakes. If you eat later than 6:00 p.m., keep meals simple. Do not forget to consume high carbohydrate foods after exercise such as bananas, yogurt, raisins, and orange juice.

One to three days prior to the marathon you need to hydrate well before the race. Your race day performance depends largely on how much water and other fluids you drink several days in advance of the race. If you're drinking enough water and other fluids your urine should be clear by 3:00 to 6:00 p.m. the day before the race.

Your daily food intake should consist of 60-70 percent carbohydrates, 15 percent protein, and twenty to twenty-five percent fat about three days before the event. Try to eat well the day before the race and plan your evening and pre-race meal to allow food enough time to digest. Some general rules to follow is to allow three to four hours for large meals to digest; two to three hours for a smaller meal; one to two hours for blended or liquid meals; and less than an hour for a snack. Finally, cut your toenails short to reduce friction inside your shoes.

LIST OF ITEMS YOU WANT TO BE PREPARED FOR BEFORE THE START OF A MARATHON

There are definitely last-minute preparations that one needs to be prepared for before the start of a marathon event so provided is a list to keep in mind:

1. Set out your entire marathon package the night before including your shoes, socks, shorts, shirt (Bib number pinned on it)

2. Make sure to put your chip in your shoes the night before, so that way you won't forget it.

3. When getting sleep, it's actually two nights before the marathon that you need to get your best night's sleep. More than likely, you will be somewhat restless the night before the marathon and will not get your best rest, so the night before that is the best night for rest.

4. Make sure you actually eat the food/drink about one and a half to two hours before the start of the run. That way you won't have a heavy feeling in your stomach before the run.

5. Upon completion of the marathon, stretch immediately. Hold the stretches for a minimum of twenty to thirty seconds.

6. Even though you are tired after the marathon try not to sit or lay down. By doing this, you can avoid heavy stiffness the day after the marathon.

FACTS ABOUT CARBO-LOADING

Are some carbohydrates better than others? Studies have shown that high glycemic carbohydrates like potatoes, rice, and pasta give you a quick rise in glucose whereas low glycemic carbohydrates like beans, whole grains, give you glucose in a slow, time released way. You do not have to be worried about gaining weight from carbo loading. You may add two to four pounds of water weight before your running competition, but this actually means your carbo loading has worked. The water will be released and used during the race.

Furthermore, stocking up on carbohydrates, you need to remember to load up on water until about two hours before your race and on race day, eat a good breakfast that will give you energy. It's recommended best to eat a high carbohydrate diet every day and this will keep your muscles well fueled and will allow you to train hard. Carbohydrate loading incorporated before running competition is like adding extra fuel to your tank that will certainly help your race performance.

TWO REASONS THE LONG RUN IS SO IMPORTANT

It's very fitting what Lori Culnane said: "Everything you ever wanted to know about yourself, you can learn in 26.2 miles." The most important workout for full marathon runners is the once-a-week long run. First time marathoners should be up to twelve miles on their long run and experienced runners aiming to break three hours should be up to fourteen to sixteen miles before gradually increasing their mileage toward their longest long run of the year aiming at twenty miles. Two reasons the long run is so important.

Number one, it simulates the distance you're running the best and you're spending more time on your feet, and the second reason is that's where you gain the most confidence. You're building longer mileage, so you're gaining more and more confidence. Due to the long run being so important, beginning marathoners should rest the day before and stay off their feet as much as possible. The second most important work out of the week is the recovery day after the long run and it's recommended that people cross-train that day by walking, cycling, or swimming for forty-five to sixty minutes. You beat yourself up a little bit on the long run and you're tired and you're sore. Something light, swimming or cycling, loosens you up a little better and mentally (because you're doing something other than running), you're getting a little refreshed.

People should be running a minimum of four times a week and preferably five, and runners should also be stretching after workouts, using the foam roller and paying special attention to the hips and the iliotibial band, the fibers that run along the outside of the leg. You should drink plenty of water throughout the week and generally runners don't drink enough water.

MARATHON TRAINING PHYSIOLOGICAL BENEFITS

Running 26.2 miles is no small feat. In fact, it is an amazing physical and psychological goal and achievement. No other sport is so popular and yet so physically demanding as marathon running. Nevertheless, studies show that the physiological benefits far outweigh the physical stresses of marathon running. While running a marathon is very hard, our bodies do a miraculous job of recovering and repairing itself. Once physical aches and pains subside, you'll come away with stronger bones, heart, and muscles.

What is more powerful and beneficial than the physical gains are the psychological and emotional benefits. Every runner who sets goals, trains for, and accomplishes those goals has accomplished something remarkable.

As a running coach who has provided guidance to thousands of runners over the course of twenty-six years, I can attest that completing a marathon can be a life changing event and accomplishment. Only 1 percent of the world's population can say they are a marathoner. So, if you are part of this elite group of people, you should be very proud.

GLYCOGEN DEPLETION FACTORS

Carbohydrate-loading dinners have become a staple of the modern marathon prerace events. Carbohydrate loading makes sense and for example, carbohydrates provide energy to the muscles faster than fats and are required for optimal aerobic performances. Carbohydrate loading does improve performance in endurance sports lasting longer than ninety minutes. While carbohydrate loading does appear to be effective for most runners, it does have its drawbacks. Consuming too many calories in the name of carbohydrate loading can add extra body weight which will increase the energy demands of running a marathon. For every three grams of water are stored with it, and this can leave a runner with a bloated or heavy feeling.

Some experts feel that consuming carbohydrates during a marathon is just as important if not more so as carbohydrate loading. Studies show the importance of carbohydrate as a fuel source during prolonged running but the issue of when and how much carbohydrate should be consumed seems to be an individual matter. Carbohydrate loading starts with three days of a low carbohydrate diet followed by intense exercise to deplete glycogen stores. This is followed by three days of high carbohydrate consuming. Carbohydrates during a marathon should be done at a rate of 120 to 180 calories per hour and thirty to forty minutes prior to fatigue. It's up to the individual to determine whether sport drinks, energy gels, bananas, or some other type of carbohydrate works best.

MARATHON EFFECTS ON YOUR BODY

Running a marathon has been viewed by some experts as too extreme to be healthy so provided are two physiological stresses of running a marathon:

1. The major cause of hyponatremia, or low blood sodium levels, is drinking too much water which dilutes sodium levels in the blood. Low sodium levels cause swelling or edema in the brain. The best way to prevent this serious problem is to drink in moderation before and during a marathon. Common recommendations for marathon runners are to drink twenty ounces of fluid two to three hours before the race and another eight ounces thirty minutes before. During the marathon, runners should switch between drinking eight to ten ounces of water, and it's recommended consuming an electrolyte at most of the aid stations throughout the race. This can be done by taking in a sport drink every ten to twenty minutes and afterward drink as much as they comfortably can.

2. Hypothermia can be the main environmental concern for marathon runners. The risk for hypothermia is greater in cold, windy, or wet weather; however, the American College of Sports Medicine cites other factors that may reduce body temperature. If the second half of the marathon is run slower than the first half, not enough heat may be generated to maintain body temperature. Furthermore, any sweat that builds up can saturate clothing, which will draw additional heat away from the body. Hypothermia can also occur after the race when heat radiates from a warm body to the cooler air temperature. It's recommended to prevent hypothermia by dressing in layers, with an outer layer that protects from wind and water. Layers should be removed as air temperature increases to avoid hyperthermia and any wet layers should be replaced.

TAPERING FOR THE MARATHON/HALF MARATHON DISTANCE

For everyone who prepares for the marathon or half marathon distance, your taper period will need to be longer, so provided are recommendations on tapering. A month before the big race you need to cut back using a 75-50-30-15 plan. That is, do 75 percent of usual mileage the first week, 50 percent the second week and so on. For a half marathon then you need to take on a two-week 50-15 plan.

During the initial three weeks of the marathon/half marathon taper, do your hard workouts as you have been, but reduce the easy miles. During the last week, emphasize interval work; equally divide between 5K race pace and marathon race pace. Be sure you have done some of these workouts in the weeks leading up to your taper so these taper workouts will not make you sore.

Like all proven training schedules, tapering is a combination of work and rest. It allows your muscles to recover and rebuild after periods of hard work. Tapering produces an incredible array of changes, including greater muscle glycogen stores, expanded blood plasma, increased aerobic enzymes, improved running economy, and heightened mental freshness.

MARATHON TRAINING INJURY CONCERNS

While attending a marathon clinic a few years ago, the presenting clinician informed everyone in attendance that it takes between 30,000 and 50,000 steps to run a marathon. Every time the foot hits the ground, a stress three to four times your body weight is absorbed by the ankles, knees, hips, and lower back. Furthermore, with each stride, some muscles contract to propel the body forward while others control the degree of movement by being lengthened. The lengthening or eccentric contractions are notorious for damaging the muscles infrastructure. As a result, muscle damage and inflammation can remain for seven days after finishing running a marathon, while repair of muscle fibers can take three to twelve weeks.

Fortunately, only a relatively few marathon runners have experienced injuries while running a marathon that caused them to seek medical attention. While muscle soreness is the major health issue for the average marathon runner, elite runners have additional concerns. Some of the factors that increase the risk for injury while running a marathon are running a first marathon, participation in other sports, illness during the two weeks prior, current use of medication, and training mileage. My experience has shown that runners who train less than forty-five miles per week were more likely to become injured while running a marathon. The primary reason for this is that runners might be doing too much too quickly during the marathon due to the fact they did not acquire the suitable amount of mileage during training.

Higher levels of training have been shown to decrease the risk for knee injuries but increase the risk of injury to the quadriceps and hamstrings during a marathon. With the large number of training miles required to prepare for running a marathon, it is not surprising that 29 to 43 percent of runners develop injuries during training. In fact, the number of injuries from running a marathon is five to ten times less than while training for a marathon. The pre-marathon injury rate increases with the number of training miles run per week with most injuries occurring to the feet and knees followed by shins and hips.

"The strongest people aren't the people who win, but the people who don't give up when they lose."

— Liam Payne

RACE DAY
PERFORMANCE TIPS

MARATHON RUNNING TIPS

Susan Sidoriak said it best: "*I dare you to train and race a marathon and not have it change your life.*" Below are ten recommendations for a successful race:

1. Start slow: Your pace the first three to four miles should be thirty to forty-five seconds slower than your overall marathon pace.

2. Friday, two days before the race if your marathon is on a Sunday, is the most important night's sleep.

3. Do not spend too much time at the expo so you can stay off your feet.

4. The day before the race set out your entire marathon package including shoes, shorts, shirt, timing chip and bib number.

5. Don't do anything new on race day. No experimenting.

6. Drive the course to familiarize yourself with the route.

7. Stay hydrated before, during and after the race.

8. Drink at all the aid stations but don't stop moving.

9. Try to not think of the finish line. It's recommended that you break the race into different parts of the 26.2-mile distance.

10. Upon finishing the race, stretch immediately and keep moving for at least twenty minutes. Perhaps spin very easy on a stationary bike for twenty to thirty minutes a few hours after the marathon.

MARATHON RACE DAY PLAN & APPROACH TO THE 26.2 MILE DISTANCE

This scripture passage by Ecclesiastes serves as a powerful reminder for us all that *"If you ever wait for perfect conditions, you'll never get anything done."* Subsequently, success in the marathon distance can be achieved from these provided four steps:

Pre-race execution: You need to carry out everything you've planned and do not spend any energy doing unnecessary things. The expo being the day before the race, you need to just get your number and go back home. Do not stand on your feet all day and sit whenever you have the opportunity. On race morning, drink liquids before the race.

Controlled start: Go out slower than what you want to average and stay relaxed. Enjoy the spectators and if you run the first mile too fast then slow it down. It's recommended you run thirty seconds off your final average pace at the start and monitor yourself through those early miles and take in liquids including water and electrolytes at every mile.

Race begins: After six to eight miles, it is time to start running below average pace to make up for the slower early miles. You have some time to make up, but you do not have to make it up immediately. Still try to run relaxed and relax your shoulders. At Mile 20, the race begins. You are now tired, but if you have been in control throughout the race, you know you can do it. Time to focus. All that running has to come into fruition these last few miles. Do not back off the intensity because it hurts. You spent too much time preparing for this so run as fast as your legs can carry you the last four to six miles of the marathon.

Exquisite pain: If you can do the above, then at Mile 24 the pain will become exquisite. What that means is that you are going to finish, and you are going to finish strong. You are going to pass people, taking in the applause of the spectators and gaining energy with every step. It's exhilarating.

HYPERTHERMIA HEALTH CONCERN

Running marathons can create issues and be problematic for a few athletes with respect to hyperthermia. Besides supplying oxygen-rich blood to the body, the heart helps control body temperature by pumping warm blood to the skin where body heat is lost through the evaporation of sweat.

During a marathon, heat loss and production can increase over ten-fold. High humidity and dehydration can make heat loss more difficult. High humidity levels reduce evaporation, while dehydration impairs the ability to transfer heat from the muscles to the skin. Either situation will increase body temperature and risk heat issues for runners. Muscle weakness and disorientation can develop with body temperature of 105-106 degrees Fahrenheit and a loss of consciousness can occur with body temperature near 107 degrees Fahrenheit. Without the ability to lose heat through evaporation, body temperature would rise fast enough to cause heat problems after only fifteen to twenty minutes of running. Even with the ability to sweat, it is not uncommon for marathon runners to finish the 26.2 miles with body temperature of 105 degrees Fahrenheit.

Since dehydration reduces the amount of blood available for heat removal, one way to prevent hyperthermia would be to drink as much water as is lost through the sweat. The average sweat rate for runners is 1.2 liters per hour. Moreover, most runners either can't tolerate drinking that much or choose not to drink that much liquid. Typically, runners drink as little as 200 milliliters per hour but rarely more than one liter per hour. Therefore, it is not uncommon for runners to lose two to ten percent of their body weight through sweating.

POST-MARATHON WORKOUTS

Post-marathon recovery is one very important aspect of training that's frequently overlooked. Very often the effects of recovery leave runners feeling mentally and physically flat for weeks. An ideal recovery plan provides needed rest in a carried twenty-eight-day schedule that will get you in great shape within the month. It's important during the first week of the plan that you completely stop training. Whether you reached your goal or not, don't run a step that week! Since running a marathon depletes your body's energy stress along with causing some muscle tissue damage, resting from training will help your body to rebuild.

However, it's recommended that you spin lightly on a stationary bike for thirty minutes every other day; such a workout will improve your circulation and flexibility. During the week you should also replenish carbohydrates and drink several eight-ounce glasses of water daily. During week two you can begin easy running again and about ten days after the race you should do a tempo run. A tempo run will boost your fitness, but it won't further stress your still tired muscles the way an interval workout would do. If you ran the marathon on a Sunday, you should do the tempo run ten days later on a Wednesday. Warm-up slowly and thoroughly for ten minutes, then run for twenty minutes at a pace twenty seconds faster than your marathon speed you just executed. Follow up with a ten-minute cool down. On the fourteenth day after the marathon, repeat the workout. Run very easily (twenty to thirty minutes) on the other days of the second week. Try not to be afraid to take complete days off. Your mileage that second week should be 25 percent of your usual marathon-training mileage.

In week three you'll begin upgrading your aerobic capacity by running some long intervals. On the Tuesday of that week do a workout on the track or trails of 3 x 1200-meter repeats at 45 seconds per mile faster than your marathon pace. On Friday, do 3 x 1-mile intervals at the same tempo and run thirty to forty minutes on the other days. Week three mileage should be 35 percent of usual. During week four you should begin restoring some of the foot speed you may have lost during your marathon build-up. On Monday and Thursday run 8-10 X 200-meter intervals on the track, trails, or road at a pace somewhat faster than your 5K race pace. Warm-up and cool down thoroughly and jog three minutes between each hard interval. Concentrate on staying relaxed and holding your form and during the other days of the week you should run easy for forty to fifty minutes. A sensible and carefully planned recovery is the key to enjoying running again and getting yourself geared up for your next marathon!

PRE-RACE RELAXATION TECHNIQUES

It's amazing how silent all the chatter becomes when you are laser-focused on a single goal. Blood raced through my veins while my tunnel vision narrowed as I was acutely aware of my current situation; lined shoulder to shoulder amongst the top ten milers in the world to race four laps around the track at London's Crystal Palace in 1991. My heart was pounding. I took a deep breath and stepped forward, aiming to stay relaxed, and although I only heard silence, there were 20,000 screaming fans above me, but, at that moment, I was still. That past personal racing experience still resonates with me today and every long-distance runner who competes and wishes to do their best experiences pre-race jitters, which can cause butterflies in the stomach and heaviness in the legs. It's important to realize that pre-race nervousness is good. It means you care about your upcoming performance. Your pulse as you are walking around should be between 100 and 110 HR. If it's higher, it's recommended trying some relaxation techniques so provided are a few recommendations.

In the hours and minutes before the race, visualize yourself running smooth, strong, and relaxed. Focus more on how you will run the race than on what the outcome will be. Reassure yourself that you have done the training, you are prepared, and you are ready to race. Try repeating affirmations such as "I may or may not win, but I belong here" or "I have trained well for this race, once it starts, I will feel fine." If you still feel overly anxious, take some slow, deep breaths in through the nose and out through the mouth.

It's also recommended you record in your training log how you feel before and during your races. Over time, you may notice a pattern emerging as to what emotions helped produce your best performances. Try to recreate that emotional state before your upcoming races. If pre-race nervousness is a serious problem for you. the recommendation is to see a sports psychologist.

VISUALIZATION IS HELPFUL TOOL IN CROSS-COUNTRY RACES

For the sport of Cross-Country, individual preparation entails that you work on the mental and physical realm always. In particular, the type of mental training technique that runners can practice individually is visualization. At San Diego State University, our Cross-Country team would engage in the practice of visualization every day, and this was one of the primary reasons we were ranked 14th in the nation during my senior year in 1987.

Visualization or thinking through a cross-country course or track race prior to the event is critical for your success. When practiced regularly, visualization can be one of the most effective training techniques for improving athletic performance. Early in my running career, I set a personal goal of breaking four minutes in the mile, and I suppose the sub-four-minute mile has always intrigued humanity since we can relate to the subtleties of it all. One runs four laps in under four minutes. The mental preparation involved in the pursuit of my sub-four-minute mile goal began when I was a freshman in high school and this is when I wrote down on a piece of paper the split times I needed to run.

Every day I would look at those splits and visualize achieving my goal; the splits were 60, 60, 60, and 59 and the visualization practice worked. On June 10th, 1989, I ran the one-mile in 3:59.79 and officially became the 168th American to run a sub-four-minute mile. Picturing a successful performance builds pre-race confidence and helps runners identify and overcome possible race day obstacles. While physical training is still very important, mental training and visualization are meant to train our minds and create neural patterns in our brains to help our muscles do exactly what we want them to do with precision and perfection.

The last two miles of a cross-country race, when the runner begins to fatigue, are the most important mentally. If a runner is tiring, he/she should single out a competitor he or she thinks they can catch, gradually work up to that runner, and then hang behind before you go past your competitor. You need to focus on your form and on feeling powerful, then return to your original pace and set up another target to pass. A runner who is being pursued in a race must think positively and he or she must tell themselves they're strong, powerful, and ready for the competition. When the runner hears a competitor approaching from behind, he or she should try to prevent the other runner from passing and maintain contact as long as possible. Maintaining this contact, staying within five to ten yards, will give your mind something to do besides get mad or nervous and it allows you to keep engaged in the race.

"Strength doesn't come from what you can do; it comes from overcoming the things you once thought you couldn't."

— Rikki Rogers

TIPS FOR PREVENTION AND TREATMENT OF COMMON AILMENTS

SOURCES OF FATIGUE

Curing fatigue could be as simple as getting more sleep. Working long hours plus training hard may mean you lack time to rest adequately. You may have to restructure your schedule to let time for sleep become more of a priority.

It's important to set aside time on the weekends to sleep in so that you can prepare yourself for another busy week. Some people miss out on sleep because they overeat at dinner and consequently have trouble falling asleep. If this is your cause, try eating smaller dinners but bigger breakfasts. Over the years I have experienced the same struggles. A heartier breakfast will not only curb your desire to overeat at night but also boost your morning blood sugar and fuel your muscles for more energy during the day.

Mental fatigue along with physical fatigue can slow you down. If you are undergoing a major life change such as divorce, new job, death of a friend or relative, you may be expending a lot of energy to cope with this major adjustment due to stress. If you allow more time for sleep and if you eat regularly scheduled wholesome meals, your body will have a better chance of coping. By making healthful dietary choices, you'll feel better emotionally and physically. My experience is that people hear what they want to hear, so runner's experiences and beliefs determine what they hear especially in terms of acquiring more sleep.

WAYS TO AVOID OVERTRAINING

Toward the end of my racing career, I personally suffered from this condition called overtraining and this largely contributed to why I retired from competition. Overtraining is real, so no matter what your weekly mileage, you can make the most of your workouts by following these recommendations:

1. Eat more carbohydrates a few days before increasing training duration or intensity.

2. During days of heavy training, eat a diet that's 70 percent carbohydrate calories. This amounts to approximately three to four grams of carbohydrate for every pound of body weight.

3. Although hard training may reduce your appetite, make the effort to reach for high-carbohydrate foods, especially in the first hour after your workout. I recommend keeping fruit, quick cook rice, tortillas, whole grain bread, and carbohydrate beverages handy.

4. Monitor your resting heart rate for signs of overtraining. Check your pulse before you get out of bed in the morning. If it's five to ten beats per minute above your normal resting pulse, you need a rest day.

5. Don't ignore other signs that may indicate you are overdoing it, especially mood changes, irritability, lack of appetite, and decreased sexual drive.

6. Make sleep a priority, especially during heavy training. Aim for seven to eight hours a night.

AVOIDING THE OVERTRAINING BLUES

My competitive running career ended abruptly in 1996 and this was due to overtraining and this condition affected me personally as an individual. The noticeable signs that I overtrained included fatigue, stale training, poor race performance, irritability, and an overall loss of enthusiasm for running, and this was caused by excessive mileage and too many consecutive harder workouts a year earlier in 1995.

Serious overtraining can cause sleep disturbances, hampered immune function, poor appetite, and in women, the cessation of menstrual periods. For solutions to this issue, I highly recommend one needs to cut back on their running for a minimum of two weeks. My recommendation includes experimenting with cutting back on mileage, adding rest days, and substituting cross-training days to see what works best.

If you suspect serious overtraining, just know your running form can return to normal provided you cut your running back to only two to three days a week, thirty to forty-five minutes at an easy to moderate effort. You can supplement this with more stretching and some cross-training on other days of the week, but no more than an hour at an easy to moderate effort. This will take time and patience on your part in the days and weeks ahead.

When you're feeling better, and you are ready to increase your running, then it's encouraged to continue monitoring your resting heart rate in the morning and look at your training over a year and plan periods when you will train hard and race. After that follow these periods of easier running and lower mileage.

OVERTRAINING SIGNS

Many athletes experience heavy legs and lackluster performances during periods of increased training. While increased training generally improves performance, there is a point at which an athlete's body becomes overburdened. The first and most obvious sign of overtraining is a noticeable drop in performance.

Signs of overtraining include consistent days of a higher resting heart rate, especially in the morning. Other symptoms like fatigue, moodiness, irritability, and even a lower sex drive can be difficult to connect to overtraining, but nonetheless it does have an impact. One of the primary factors in these negative effects on the body may be diet, and studies suggest that runners who train heavily and skip on daily carbohydrate intake can lose some of the benefits of hard training. It's critical to review periodically your entire training plan to determine if there are any weaknesses and needed improvements. In many instances overtraining is worse than some more serious running injuries due to the fact it takes much longer to overcome the overtraining blues. My personal experience with overtraining led me to never being able to return back to maximum form again. Be careful and be mindful every day.

HOW TO REMEDY SIDE STICHES?

Every runner will experience side stiches during their running career and certainly it was one of the most frustrating ailments for me over the years. A side stich is a sharp pain that usually is felt just below the rib cage and is caused by a cramp in the diaphragm, gas in the intestines, or food in the stomach. Stiches normally come on during harder workouts.

If you get a stitch on your right side which is more common, slow down for thirty seconds and exhale forcefully each time your left foot hits the ground. If the stitch is on the left, exhale hard when your right foot lands. Continue until pain recedes. If this does not help, try slow, deep "belly breathing." This means your abdomen should go in and out with each breath. I also recommend you run with hands on top of your head and your elbows back while you breathe deeply from your belly.

Another remedy is to take your fist and dig it under your ribcage, push the fist in with your other arm and bend your torso over to ninety degrees. I recommend you run like this for ten steps; this in effect stretches the diaphragm, and most stitches are caused by a spasm of the diaphragm. If none of these techniques work, stop and walk until the pain subsides. Finally, to prevent stitches caused by food in the stomach, don't eat less than an hour before you run.

PREVENTING AND TREATING FOOT PROBLEMS

The most effective path to healthy feet begins with common sense. This not only can help prevent foot problems from occurring but also will help with treatment when problems arise. Below are five ways to prevent foot problems.

1. Do not ignore foot pain as pain is not normal. Runners who suffer from foot pain should see a podiatrist.

2. Poorly fitting shoes are thought to be the primary cause of 80 percent of all foot problems.

3. Check your shoe size periodically because the feet continue to grow longer and wider as individuals age. It's recommended you check your shoe size at least once every three years.

4. Losing weight can help against possible foot problems. The lighter an individual is, the less force has to be dispersed since the feet and ankles serve as shock absorbers.

5. When running, wear shoes that have good arch support and proper cushioning with an appropriate amount of space in the forefoot. Proper fit in your shoes is important.

MASSAGE HELPS PREVENT INJURIES AND MAY IMPROVE YOUR PERFORMANCE

Massage therapy is the hands-on manipulation of the soft tissues of the body, which are the muscles, fascia, tendons, and ligaments. It involves moving and applying pressure to these tissues. The three types of massage beneficial to runners include Swedish massage, which is gentle and relaxing, and sports massage, which focuses on muscle groups relevant to a particular sport. The third type is pressure point therapy, which is used primarily for injury treatment.

Massage can definitely improve the functioning of the circulatory, lymphatic, musculoskeletal, and nervous systems and it enhances the rate at which the body recovers from injury, illness or even more a hard training or racing effort. Massage stretches the muscles, moving fluids to remove wastes and improve circulation. Massage therapy also dissolves what is called knots which are really muscle fibers and connective tissues that have adhered to each other. Massage therapy is highly recommended for both injury prevention and may even improve your race performances. For the past thirty-five years, I have received massage therapy sessions once a week and have experienced tremendous benefits from Swedish and sports massage along with pressure point therapy.

COLD TREATMENT BENEFITS FOR INJURIES

Most often when you have an injury, tissue is stretched and torn, and swelling occurs. Swelling interferes with healing so anything that will prevent or reduce swelling should help you recover from a minor injury more quickly. The sooner you attend to swelling after an injury the better, and the best approach is to apply cold treatment directly to the injured area immediately.

In essence, cold therapy shrinks the blood vessels, which reduces bleeding in the area and helps to prevent swelling. Cold therapy also prevents the muscles from going into spasm, which are involuntary contractions, and relieves pain. The use of cold treatment is as old as the practice of medicine. When you apply cold, the skin will initially feel cold, often followed by relief of pain from the injury. As icing progresses, you will feel a burning sensation, then pain in the skin, and finally numbness.

It is believed too much cold for too long can cause frostbite or even nerve damage, so the length of time you apply cold will vary depending on the method and location of the injury. Areas with little body fat like the knee or ankle do not tolerate cold as well as fatty areas like the thigh and buttocks. For best results, it's recommended to apply cold therapy at regular intervals throughout the waking hours of the day, allowing a few hours between treatments. The time off from cold treatment will keep cooling effects from accumulating and will allow the skin to return to normal temperature. An ice bag remains the cold treatment of choice for most athletes, but several options do exist.

Over the years I have also advised hundreds of runners after a longer run to jump into the ocean and bathe their legs for twenty minutes in the water. The water temperature of the Pacific Ocean averages 57 to 60 degrees which are similar temperatures to an indoor whirlpool. I call this practice utilizing the ocean as a God-made ice whirlpool.

THE USE OF ICE BAGS FOR INJURY TREATMENT

Ice bags are for applying deep, penetrating cold. You simply fill a bag made of thick plastic, rubber, or moisture-proof fabric with ice and apply it directly to the skin. The cooling effect of ice bags lasts long and is more effective than some of the superficial methods like ice massage. If you use a regular plastic food bag, then it's recommended you place a thin towel like a dish towel between the bag and your skin.

A shortcoming to ice bags is getting the bag to contour to the curves of the body for maximum application. The bag will mold better if you don't fill it completely with ice or if you use crushed ice. An alternative is to use a bag of frozen peas or corn. The bag will conform nicely to the injured part of the body, and it's suggested you place a thin towel between the bag and the skin.

The time recommendation to apply ice bags to an injury area is twenty minutes depending on the body part and comfort.

WHEN TO AVOID COLD THERAPY

Using cold therapy may not be a good idea for some people. Those who are very sensitive to cold will not be able to tolerate icing long enough to do any good. Conversely, those who have a high tolerance to cold or who pride themselves on "being tough" regarding injuries might apply cold therapy too long. People with problems in the blood vessels near the skin should avoid cold therapy, especially those with Raynaud's phenomenon (a condition in which the blood vessels in the fingers, toes, ears, and nose constrict dramatically when exposed to cold and other stimuli).

If you suspect you may be at risk because of diabetes or another condition that can diminish blood flow, then it's recommended checking with your doctor before applying ice to an injury if you happen to fall under this condition.

THE ROLE HEAT HAS ON INJURY TREATMENT

Most runners might not realize this but heat, like ice, can deaden pain, and many people will attest that it feels good. The problem is that it can also promote swelling, which is something you want to avoid after an injury, Furthermore, heat may increase deep circulation, which can be devastating if bleeding is involved. As a running coach, I rarely prescribe heat to my runners for injury treatment for these same reasons mentioned.

Once the injury is under control, and your greatest discomfort is associated with stiffness, heat can help. Usually this means at least two to three days after the injury occurred. You can use hot packs or a hot bath and/or jacuzzi to help loosen up the joint before activity. It's recommended one needs to be very careful of developing any swelling so if this happens you must stay away from the heat.

THE PREVENTION AND TREATMENT OF HAMMERTOES

Hammertoes are a deformity of a toe resulting in a widened, buckled-under hammerhead shape, often due to repeated rubbing against the front of the running shoe. As for treatment be sure your running shoes are roomy enough in the toe box. Apply a doughnut pad to the top of the affected toe to reduce friction and pain. It's recommended you stretch out the toe as often as possible and some runners have luck taping the affected toe to an adjacent toe or toes to keep it from worsening. Athletes with big hammertoes may want to use running shoes for their everyday wear.

This condition of hammertoes usually occurs in the second, third, or fourth toe. The toe is bent or contracted. Furthermore, the little toe is usually curved. Hammertoes are not painful themselves; however, they rub against your shoes and the friction and pressure can create a buildup of hard thick tissue which can be very painful.

Hammertoes result from a misalignment of the foot. The condition may be inherited, but usually excessive over pronation causes the tendons of the toe to pull at a strange angle, making the toe bend. Gradually, the toe gets fixed in a bent position and a buildup of tissue develops to protect the toe joint where it rubs against your shoe. Making this condition even worse are ill-fitting running shoes that rub against the toes. As for the prevention of hammertoes, motion control shoes reduce over-pronation as do orthotics. In any event, make certain your running shoes are wide enough in the forefoot to prevent rubbing and the formation of thick tissue.

It's best to catch the condition of hammertoes in its early stages before the toe becomes fixed. Orthotic devices or arch supports can correct the biomechanical problem causing the hammertoe. For example, you can also try an over-the-counter device called a hammertoe crest pad, which will help move your toe back into a normal position. Reduce the hard tissue with an emery board or sandpaper. If the tissue becomes too painful, then cover them with moleskin. If your toe is in a fixed position, you either have to put up with the pain or undergo surgery to correct the contracted joint. You can continue running with this injury provided it's not too painful or you are not favoring it in any way.

THE PREVENTION AND TREATMENT OF CHAFING

Long-distance runners often suffer from chafing. Many of my marathoners in particular seem to experience this condition more as they experience painful skin irritation caused by friction. It's recommended you need to remove the source of friction by trying different clothing in different cuts or different fibers. To prevent this problem, you need to avoid cotton because it stays wet. Synthetics are better. For chafed thighs, short Lycra tights may minimize friction. Women whose sports bras may cause chafing should look for one with flat or covered seams.

To treat chafing, one needs to apply petroleum jelly or talcum powder to the sensitive areas to prevent further irritation or cover the chafed spot with a bandage. When your nipples are rubbing try a product called "Corn Cushions" which offer good protection from friction and peel off easily after your run.

SHOULD I RUN WITH BACK PAIN?

Pain or aching in the back may have any one of several causes. If running doesn't make it worse you are free to run; however, sitting can place more stress on the back than running does on the body. It's recommended that exercise rather than rest is best for most people with back problems. If running is not comfortable than perhaps you can swim, cycle, or try some other activity. Walking is an excellent exercise in this case.

For back pain relief, always use ice, but rather than wrap the ice against your back, place it on your bed and lie on it. If necessary, use pillows if you're too uncomfortable. Some people favor a hot/cold regimen from the beginning. It's recommended you alternate twenty minutes of ice with twenty minutes of heat. To be honest, some back problems lie deep in the muscles, where icing will not have an effect. If pushing the site of the injury with your thumb does not cause pain, the injury probably lies too deep.

People with chronic back problems should do stretching and strengthening exercises regularly. It's recommended you try back extensions, lower back stretches, pelvic tilts, bent leg crunches, and trunk twists provided there is no discomfort. Make sure you warm up beforehand. When running, stick to soft surfaces and avoid irregular surfaces, hills, and small running areas with tight turns. When you sleep, place a pillow between your knees when on your side; add two pillows under your knees when lying on your back. Finally, if your back pain radiates into your leg or if rest and home treatments don't bring relief, then it's time to see a doctor.

EXERCISES TO PREVENT AND TREAT LOW BACK PAIN

There are six exercises that you can do to prevent and treat low back pain. Many of my athletes often complain about low back pain due to the high impact running has on the body and the hard surfaces they run on. These exercises below help provide for a flexible lumbar spine and strong abdominal muscles, which are both important for preventing and alleviating low back pain. It's recommended you perform these exercises daily and hold each stretch for twenty to thirty seconds at a time.

1. **Pelvic tilt:** Lie on your back with knees bent, feet flat on the floor, and arms at your sides. Tighten your stomach muscles and flatten the small of your back against the floor, without pushing down with the legs. Hold for five seconds, then slowly relax.

2. **Knee to shoulder:** Starting in the same position as for the pelvic tilt, grasp your right knee and gently pull it toward your right shoulder. Return to the starting position and repeat with the left leg.

3. **Double knee to chest:** Starting in the same position as for the pelvic tilt, grasp your right leg and pull it close to your chest, and then pull the left leg even with the right. Pull both knees toward your shoulders. Let your knees return to arm's length and repeat.

4. **Hamstring Stretch:** From the same starting position as in the pelvic tilt, bring one knee to your chest and then straighten the leg, stretching the heel toward the ceiling. You should feel the stretch behind your knee. Bend the knee and return the leg to the starting position. Repeat with the other leg.

5. **Trunk Flexion, prone:** Starting on your hand and knees, tuck in your chin and arch your back, and then slowly sit back on your heels

while lowering your shoulders to the floor. Relax. Return to the starting position, keeping stomach tight and back arched.

6. **Trunk Flexion, seated:** Sitting near the edge of a chair, spread legs apart and cross arms over your chest. Be sure the chair will not slip backward or tip. Tuck your chin and slowly curl your trunk downward. Relax. Uncurl slowly into an upright position, raising your head last.

STRUGGLING WITH CALCANEAL BUMPS

The bony protuberance behind the heel is a condition known as calcaneal bump. Most often associated with a high arched foot, the bony prominence pushes into the back heel counter of your shoe. Both the tendon and the soft tissues can become inflamed and painful when this occurs. If you have arched foot, the heel bone (calcaneus) can change alignment and this causes an enlargement of the bone will create a bursa, which is a sack of fluid that protects your tendon and other soft tissues. When you're wearing shoes, this bursa gets pushed up against the heel counter and becomes painful. Without proper diagnosis, and if you recognize you have a high arched foot, it's important to wear a well-cushioned shoe that will not have an overly firm heel counter.

For treatment it has been suggested cutting away the heel area of your shoes to minimize pressure against the protuberance. Another alternative is to cut a doughnut shape from a piece of moleskin to place around the bump. If these methods don't work, then you might want to see a podiatrist. A podiatrist or orthopedic surgeon may inject the bursa with cortisone to reduce the inflammation or prescribe their patient wearing an immobilizer boot to reduce the pressure. In some more severe cases the podiatrist may suggest surgery since this might be required to shave off the bone spur so that the patient can return to normal activities without pain. My own struggles with calcaneal bumps for several years ultimately led to undergoing surgery myself to rectify this issue. Although I was restricted to wearing an immobilizer boot and bearing weight of any kind for twelve weeks post-surgery, I resumed running with no pain for several years later.

PREVENTION AND TREATMENT OF ATHLETE'S FOOT

This fungal infection usually shows up under the arch of the foot or between the toes, where moisture is highest. It produces red, itchy lesions. Fortunately, the fungus lives on the outer layers of skin and will not invade your system. Moreover, constant scratching can cause a break in the skin and lead to an infection that could invade your body.

Experts do not know why one person gets the fungus and another doesn't, but athlete's foot is picked up in wet public areas such as locker rooms and swimming pools. Another equally common cause is wearing damp, dirty socks and shoes, which are prime breeding grounds for fungus. Athlete's foot can be treated with over-the-counter medications. Creams, sprays, and powders are much less effective than ointments and gels. Most people apply the medication for a few days until the symptoms are gone, but to truly eliminate this fungus, you must continue to apply the medication for two weeks after redness and itching have disappeared. Soaking your feet in baking soda mixed water also works too.

Preventative methods include wearing clean dry socks when you run. It's recommended you use over the counter foot powders and sprays to keep your feet dry. Wear sandals in showers around pools and in other wet public areas. Contrary to what many runners believe you can run with athlete's foot.

PREVENTION AND TREATMENT OF BLACK TOENAILS

A black toenail is caused by a blood blister underneath the nail. The collection of blood under the nail discolors it and can cause pressure and pain, but black toenails generally are not painful. In most cases, the toenail eventually falls off. A black toenail occurs when your toe becomes bruised from bumping against the end of your running shoe. This can happen if you do a lot of downhill running or racing or if your shoes are too small. Usually, runners with a Morton's foot type, where the second toe is longer than then the first toe, are most susceptible to having bruised second toenails.

The best way to prevent black toenails is to wear shoes that fit properly. The toe box should be wide enough and the length of the shoe long enough so your toes do not bump against the shoe. You should have about a half inch of space between the end of your longest toe and the top of your shoe. For treatment, you need to drain the blood to remove the pressure. To do this, it's recommended you swab your toenail with alcohol. Then take a paper clip or other sharp narrow object, heat it in a flame and push it through the toenail. Drain the blood, apply an antiseptic, and cover the hole with an adhesive bandage. Usually, if the toe throbs with pain, it's best to take a couple of days off from running and let the toenail heal.

SIMPLE STEPS TO KEEP YOUR KNEES HEALTHY

In my experience with coaching marathoners, knee pain is one of the more frequent injuries they experience, and runners experience various degrees of knee pain discomfort so provided are steps on preventing future problems and keeping your knees healthy.

Warm-up and stretching before running can help the knee joint by increasing the circulation of the blood and lymph fluid in and out of joint structures, ensuring your ligaments and muscles connected to your knee joint are not too tight. As a result, tension on the tendons is reduced and pressure on the knee is relieved.

Develop muscle balance by strengthening the muscles of the lower body to reduce the amount of force that goes through the knees. Make sure that you maintain an appropriate muscle balance between the quadriceps and hamstrings.

Avoiding sudden increases in the intensity of exercise will allow your body to gradually and progressively adapt to the demands that you impose on it. Running too much too soon can injure your knees. For example, running hills without a strong background may in fact increase your level of intensity and can present problems in the future.

Protecting your feet and how and where they strike the ground can have a profound effect on your knees. Two of the most meaningful actions you can undertake are to wear shoes that fit properly and provide adequate cushioning, and to immediately take care of any future foot problems.

Vary the mode of exercise: Participating in other sport activities other than running keeps you from repeatedly stressing the same bones and muscle groups, thereby keeping the stress on your knees to a minimum. For example, running stadium stairs and running downhill excessively can present knee problems.

Use exercise equipment properly: Improper use of exercise equipment can cause knee problems. If you exercise on a stationary bike for example, check the position of the pedal crank relative to the seat post. If the crank is not close to the seat post, you will place increased stress on your knees while cycling.

Keep your weight down: Maintaining on appropriate level of weight can reduce the stress on your knees. Excessive weight can increase your risk of degenerative conditions such as osteoarthritis of the knee.

Listen to your body: Pain is your body's signal that you may be placing too much stress on your knees. The primary step in ensuring that your actions don't lead to a more serious injury is by stopping whatever is causing the stress.

It's evident that utilizing prevention strategies is the key to staying consistently healthy from knee pain.

TWO EXERCISES TO KEEP YOUR KNEES HEALTHY

Pain on the outside of your knee usually means inflammation of your iliotibial band. This is properly known as iliotibial band syndrome or ITBS. This annoying condition accounts for 12 percent of all running-related overuse injuries. Research has discovered a connection between ITBS and weakness in the outer buttock muscles. To strengthen your abductors and thus decrease your risk of ITBS it's recommended trying the following two strengthening exercises below:

1. **Pelvic drops:** Stand on a step or bench, lock your knees, and lower your stronger leg off the step by shifting your weight on to your weaker leg. This should create a swivel action at the hip that lowers your foot by a couple of inches. Return to the starting position by contracting the gluteus medias. To strengthen both hip abductors, switch legs and repeat. For balance, place your hand against a wall.

2. **Side lying leg lifts:** On a padded floor or rug, lie on your side. Bend the knee of your lower leg for balance. Tighten your abdominal muscles and slightly extend your upper leg with your knee turned slightly upward. Lift your leg thirty degrees off the floor, hold for one second, and then slowly lower it.

Start with one set of fifteen to twenty repetitions and build up to thirty repetitions daily. I have seen much success with runners when these two strengthening exercises are consistently performed.

TRAINING PRINCIPLES THAT CAN PREVENT INJURIES

If your injury symptoms are severe and your injury is at an advanced stage, or if self-treatment does not seem to be working, then you need to see a sports specialist. Certainly, the best advice is not to get injured in the first place. You can help prevent injuries by following these smart training principles:

1. Wear good running shoes that fit well.

2. Replace the shoes before their midsole cushioning wears out.

3. Avoid increasing mileage by more than 10 percent a week.

4. Follow hard training days with easy days or days off running.

5. Stretch and strength train regularly.

6. When something starts to hurt, cut back or stop running until the pain is gone.

PREVENTION AND TREATMENT OF BUNIONS

A bunion is a bony growth on the side of the base of your big toe. Pressure from your shoe and motion at that joint can cause pain. Bunions gradually become worse until running and even walking are extremely painful. A bunion is an arthritic condition that can result from a genetic defect, biomechanical problems, or tight-fitting shoes so try an arch support or custom orthotic device, which will reduce over-pronation and minimize the growth of the bunion. It's recommended wearing a pad over the bunion, and cut out the area that touches the bunion. Severely disabling bunions eventually require surgery.

Assuming the condition is not inherited, the most important measure you can take from this running tip is to wear running shoes that are not too tight in the forefoot. Furthermore, if over-pronation is a problem you should wear motion control shoes. You can run with bunions unless the bunions have become too painful.

PREVENTION AND TREATMENT FOR ANKLE SPRAINS

Sprains result in pain and swelling caused by tearing or stretching of some of the ligaments surrounded the ankle, usually on the outside of the joint. As these tears heal, they form scar tissue, which sticks to normal tissue and causes inflammation and continued pain. Without appropriate treatment, ankle pain can persist for months and perhaps even years. Runners most commonly sprain ankles by stepping in a hole or tripping on a tree root or rock.

Over the years, I have experienced ankle sprains myself and there was always a risk of compensating and causing more issues elsewhere, so this is another good reason that as soon as you sprain an ankle, stop running immediately. You may feel pain right away, but your ankle can be damaged further by continuing to run so the next move you make is just as critical.

Elevate your leg and apply compression and ice. If pain and swelling persist, it's recommended you consult a doctor. A severely sprained ankle should be treated by a doctor or physical therapist who will use ultrasound and sports massage to reduce the scar tissue. If you are inclined to having ankle sprains, avoid rocky trails or any uneven terrain. Wear a firmer, more supporting training shoe for better stability and do exercises to strengthen your ankles. With respect to running with ankle sprains it's recommended no running on a sprained ankle as it will only damage it more.

TREATMENT AND PREVENTION FOR ACHILLES TENDINITIS

During my running and racing career I often ran up on my toes when executing speed workouts over track surfaces and competing in races so there were times that I personally suffered with a tight Achilles tendon. These kinds of issues are attributed to tight calf muscles, so a tight Achilles usually leads to Achilles' tendinitis and stretching the calf and tendon is imperative.

Contrary to conventional wisdom it's better to stretch your tendon after you run than before. That way, your tendon is fully warmed up and receptive to a slow gradual stretch. It's recommended to never stretch to the point of pain and consider switching to a firmer, motion control shoe to limit rear foot motion and over-pronation and make certain that there isn't any pressure or rubbing from your shoes on the Achilles tendon. One needs to eliminate or cut back on hill training.

With respect to treating the Achilles, what worked for me and what I often prescribe to athletes is taking an anti-inflammatory such as ibuprofen two or three times a day. Massage the Achilles with ice and take a few days off. In some cases, a quarter-inch to half-inch heel lift will alleviate the stress on the tendon. My recommendation is if you still have pain after a couple of weeks, you should see a sports oriented physical therapist or podiatrist.

CAN YOU RUN WITH ACHILLES TENDINITIS?

The Achilles tendon runs down the back of the leg and connects to the calf muscle. It can become inflamed from overuse and inflexibility with younger runners tend to strain the Achilles just above the heel, but as runners age, tendinitis usually occurs higher, where the Achilles connects to the calf muscle.

An inflamed Achilles feels tender and stiff. Running tends to tighten the calf muscle. When the muscle becomes too tight, it doesn't allow for the normal biomechanics of running and the Achilles tendon becomes strained and inflamed. Running steep hills or increasing your weekly mileage too quickly can lead to inflammation of the tendon. If you continue to run despite the pain, the inflammation can turn into partial tears of the tendon. Eventually, part of the tendon will die, and the weakened remaining tendon can easily rupture.

You do not want to run through Achilles' tendinitis. Even a seemingly mild Achilles' strain can turn into a partial or complete rupture, which can lead to permanent damage. Immediately beginning the therapy process will help in your recovery time with resolving this issue.

THERAPY TREATMENT FOR SHIN SPLINTS

Shin splints pain usually occurs on the inside of the shinbone caused by an overload to the shin. At times the pain radiates to the thin sheathing that surrounds the bone and sometimes to the muscle. It's recommended you treat the problem with ice and anti-inflammatories and in particular stretch the gastrocnemius calf muscle. Check if you need a new pair of shoes since that might alleviate this issue tremendously.

Another therapeutic method that worked for me during my competitive days was tapping my left foot up and down for sixty seconds followed by doing the same routine with my right foot. If you are able to run through this injury, stay away from uphill and uneven surfaces. Furthermore, the 400-meter oval track surfaces can enhance this problem too. Instead, I recommend running on a flat grassy surface that can sometimes be good, as it causes less shin twisting, and be sure to ice your shins with an ice bag for twenty minutes immediately after each run.

Stretch the calf frequently throughout the day and try using a four-inch ace bandage wrapped like a barber pole up the leg. Be sure it's not too tight for support and it's recommended you can wear it all day long but not while you sleep.

PROBLEMS WITH SUPINATION

Supination in running means insufficient inward roll of the foot after landing. Meaning, those who struggle with supination have an elevated arch and their foot rolls outward, placing extra stress on the foot. This can result in iliotibial band syndrome of the knee, Achilles' tendinitis, plantar fasciitis, and many other potential injuries. Those who have a high arch and tight Achilles tendons tend to experience supination. A tell-tale sign of a runner with supination is a shoe that is worn down on the outside edge, and if placed on a flat surface, the shoe tilts outward.

That said, shoe technology has come a long way and if you are aware of your supination, then you can proactively get gear that will help keep your supination at bay. For example, it is recommended that runners who experience supination wear shoes that help pronation (the opposite of supination). Lightweight trainers are a good option since they allow for more foot movement.

It is also recommended that supinator runners do extra stretching on calves, hamstrings, and quads. With a little extra care, you can reduce your supination tendencies and stay healthy and running strong.

SURVIVING A CALF STRAIN

In 1992, while training for the Olympic track and field trials, I suffered a calf strain that prevented me from training at 100 percent. However, with consistent physical therapy and stretching, I was able to make it to the starting line and race.

Calf strains are common, and you will likely experience some form a strain at some point in your running career. Depending on the severity of the injury, you may experience calf swelling, tenderness, and muscle tightness. Typically, a calf strain is caused by a sudden overload on the muscle from a speed workout, hill running, or uneven trails.

If you suffer from a calf strain, the best treatment is ice and anti-inflammatories. Do not try and run through the pain or stretch it out. You need to reduce swelling to promote healing. Another tip is to wrap your calf with a four-inch ace bandage. It should be tight enough to provide relief but not so tight that it cuts off circulation. Wear this all day long and during running for a couple of days. Once the swelling and pain have subsided, then you can start to gently stretch your calf five to ten times a day.

Further, you will want to lift the heel of your shoe to reduce over-extension and over-stretching when running. Try adding a quarter inch cork heel lift to your running shoes and wear street shoes with a subtle heel to reduce stress on the muscles (running shoes are often a good choice). Also avoid walking barefoot as much as possible. If you have recurring calf problems, look for shoes that are thicker in the rear foot and have a sturdy heel. With proper physical therapy and stretching, you'll be back on the roads in no time.

TREATMENT OF PLANTAR FASCIITIS

Plantar Fasciitis is pain at the base of the heel from inflammation of the plantar fascia, a band of tissue that runs from the heel to the ball of the foot. Plantar Fasciitis is a common condition affecting millions of people each year and many sufferers describe it as feeling like having a nail in your heel. Pain is usually worse in the morning or after periods of extended sitting or standing. The plantar fascia is a thick, fibrous material covering the sole of the foot that helps to balance the complex movements of the foot and ankle. It provides static support and acts as a bowstring to support the medial longitudinal arch of the foot. People who are flat-footed or whose feet roll too far inward while running or walking have a condition called over-pronation, which places stress on the plantar fascia. When the plantar fascia is stressed, it becomes inflamed and develops painful microscopic tears at the heel. These symptoms can often be reduced through the use of an orthotic, stretching, or having someone help you select a shoe that gives you support and motion control. Try different running shoes to change the pressure points and the flex of your foot.

Further suggestions on solutions to this issue are to take anti-inflammatories. Icing may not work because of the fat pad over the plantar fascia. You can give it a try by rolling your foot back and forth over a cylindrical piece of ice. This is done by using a paper cup for a mold. Stretch your calf several times a day and you can massage your foot with your hands but be cautious rubbing the tender area.

Plantar fasciitis can last from a month to a year or longer if not treated properly, and this is why an injury like this is categorized as chronic. If you cannot run without pain, then it's recommended don't and cross-train instead. If you can run, reduce your mileage. Tape the sole of your foot with one-inch athletic tape from one side of the arch to the other and consider using an arch support or heel cups. During my running and racing career I suffered from Plantar Fasciitis and was able to resolve this issue by changing the brand of shoes that I wore at the time, but obviously this remedy will not work the same for everyone.

There is always concern about heel spurs and these occur at the interface of the plantar fascia and the heel bone. At this point where ligament turns to bone, a protuberance called a tuberosity forms. Heel spurs occur naturally as we age and are not a sign of a running problem; they can only be diagnosed through an x-ray.

WHEN SHOULD YOU SEE YOUR DOCTOR IF SUFFERING FROM PLANTAR FASCIITIS?

If your foot does not feel better in a month or two it is time to visit your doctor. The following are common treatment options that are recommended for athletes who suffer from heel pain.

1. Over the counter arch supports.

2. Custom orthotics, which are inserts made from molds of your feet.

3. Oral medications such as anti-inflammatory drugs.

4. Cortisone injections.

5. Cast immobilization.

It may take nine to twelve months for your symptoms to go completely away since I have always considered plantar fasciitis a chronic problem that takes time to get over. If conservative treatment doesn't relieve your pain, although rare, surgery may be recommended. The suggestions listed above should minimize your symptoms over time and they should go away.

PLANTAR FASCIITIS THERAPY TREATMENT

You have been diagnosed with plantar fasciitis, a common cause of heel pain. This condition can develop when there is an injury or overuse of the heel bone and the band attached to it called the plantar fascia. In time, your heel pain will improve and although it may take several months, stretching and taping the foot can help in the healing process. Stretching, especially in the morning before you first get out of bed, will loosen the bottom of your foot before you step down. Stretching can help increase blood flow to the injured area, as well as increase flexibility.

The first exercise is the toe/extension stretch.

1. Before getting out of bed, pull your toes up and hold for twenty seconds.
2. Repeat these three to five times.
3. Do this stretch four times per day.

You should feel a gentle pull in the bottom of your foot. If you feel pain, let up and allow your foot to rest. If you are unable to bend over to do the stretch, ask someone else to stretch your foot. Another similar method is to use a towel to stretch your toe and foot. Furthermore, gently massage the bottom of your foot for two to three minutes to warm and loosen the sole of the foot. If you can't bend over, you can massage your foot by sitting on the side of your bed and gently rolling your foot over a tennis ball.

Unfortunately, plantar fasciitis is a difficult condition to resolve. The soleus stretch is similar to the Gastroc stretch but is done with a bent knee and targets the soleus tendon in the back of the calf. Another method you can try is to massage your foot with a frozen soda bottle. Simply put water in one-liter soda bottle and freeze it. Gently roll your foot over the bottle.

Taping the arch can also help the healing process and gives the support you need to move about more comfortably. You will need one strip of tape 1 ½ to 2 inches wide, that's long enough to wrap around your foot. Begin by placing the tape at the top of your foot and gently wrap it around the bottom of your foot. As you bring the tape around the middle of your arch, begin to pull up with some force to support the arch. Then gently wrap the tape over the top of your foot until it overlaps where the tape began.

Remember, there is a lot you can do to help your foot heal, like stretching the calf, ankle, and foot in addition to taping. By doing these things every day you will be on your way to recovery.

PREVENTION AND TREATMENT FOR BLISTERS

Blisters are caused by excess friction between running shoes and the foot. The best guarantee against blisters is a pair of shoes that fit properly. All runners should be concerned about possible blisters. They are rarely serious but can become infected and force a layoff from running if not treated properly. Fluid does accumulate between the skin's inner and outer layers due to excess friction and the cause of blisters is simply a prolonged friction between your foot, socks, and shoes.

Beginning runners sometimes get blisters because their shoes are too large. New running shoes not only need to be broken in but they also need to be kept from being broken down by use as everyday streetwear. Training shoes should be used for running only. You prevent blisters by keeping the shoes as clean and dry as possible so when shoes get wet, make sure they dry thoroughly before they are used again. It's recommended that athletes wear socks, though some runners prefer to do otherwise. Furthermore, runners should wear clean, dry socks that fit well; running without socks increases the chance of blisters, especially if the shoes get wet. When possible, leave the blister alone for twenty-four hours to allow it to heal itself. If the fluid is not reabsorbed, lance the blister as follows:

1. Sterilize a needle by heating it in a flame or boiling water or by soaking it in alcohol.

2. Swab the blister with a disinfectant such as alcohol or betadine.

3. Prick two holes on opposite sides of the blister and press gently on the blister with sterile gauze to push out the fluid. Do not remove the loose skin.

4. Smear the blister with preparation H and cover it with a sterile gauze pad. If the blister refills, lance again and then soak it in Epson salts.

Before wearing shoes, make a doughnut shape out of mole foam and place it around the blister, then put another layer on top to cover the whole area. For recurring blisters, work on eliminating the cause and make sure your running shoes are dry and before you run apply petroleum jelly or talcum powder to reduce friction. Finally, prevent infection and promote healing by applying an antibiotic ointment such as Neosporin before covering the blister with a bandage or sterile dressing.

If you are susceptible to blisters, try wearing dual-layer or blister free socks to minimize friction and moisture. Socks made from breathable synthetics work especially well to keep your feet dry. Furthermore, over the counter neoprene insoles can reduce friction. It's recommended you break in new shoes that fit properly and are correct from a biomechanical point of view since too much foot motion can cause friction. A shoe that is too tight will also cause considerable rubbing. In closing, you can run with blisters but let comfort be your guide and it's imperative to not favor your stride.

RUNNING THROUGH INJURIES

A question that's often asked is should you run with an injury? It's okay provided you run at a level below the threshold of pain. When an injury occurs, you always want to cut back your mileage and intensity until you can run without pain. It's recommended you never take medications or ice an injury before testing whether or not you can run. If it hurts no matter what, stop running and adopt a cross-training activity that includes walking, cycling, swimming, pool running, rowing, or cross-country ski machines. These activities all work with most running injuries.

If you need to stop running, take a week off and then try walk/run. If that feels okay, you can begin to return to running. If it doesn't feel good, take another week off and test your legs again. It's recommended you reintroduce yourself to running through a walk/run regimen that eventually progresses to regular steady running.

TREATMENT FOR PLANTAR WARTS

Plantar warts are hard, roundish growths that are tender to the touch and usually occur on the bottom of the feet. With your foot under a bright light, look for brownish black specs, which are indicative of plantar warts. It's recommended you sand the growth down with sandpaper or a stone and inspect it. If you see brown specs, it's a plantar wart.

For temporary relief or pain, place a doughnut-shaped piece of mole foam around the wart. To kill the wart, apply an over-the-counter liquid, gel, pad, or ointment. Be sure to follow package directions as over application of these products can burn the skin. Periodically sand and retreat the wart. It can take several months to get rid of a large one and warts can spread so monitor your feet closely and treat warts when they are small.

Another option is to apply Vitamin A once a day by breaking open a capsule and squeezing the liquid on to the wart. It can take anywhere from one to nine months for warts to disappear using this method. Remember, plantar warts thrive on moisture, so keep your feet very dry. Change your socks twice a day and apply a medicated foot powder such as Lotrimin.

GROIN PULL CAN BE PAINFUL

A pulled adductor muscle occurring suddenly during fast running, resulting in pain just below the crease between the lower abdomen and thigh, is a groin pull. Groin pain in the crease between the abdomen and thigh that develops over several weeks may indicate a stress fracture in the hip. If you believe that you are experiencing this problem, then you should see a sports physician right away.

It's recommended treating this injury with ice and anti-inflammatories and stretch. However, stretch the hamstrings first, quads secondly, and then the adductors. Wrap the area with a six-inch ace bandage and if pain persists then definitely see a sports doctor.

HAMSTRING PAIN TREATMENT

Out of all the muscle strains out there, the hamstring is the most sensitive and needy of all the muscles. Many athletes suffer from hamstring pain, including myself from time to time. And, while I have experienced many strains, I have been fortunate to have never fully pulled this muscle.

A hamstring strain manifests itself by pain in the back of the thigh and a feeling of extreme tightness. Activities that require sprinting or speed work are often the instigator. Treatment includes ice and anti-inflammatories. Most importantly, DO NOT STRETCH your hamstring! While it may seem counterintuitive, stretching worsens the tightness. Think of a rubber band — you stretch it and then it retracts. Your hamstring functions similarly. So, the best treatment is to reduce swelling and rest. Depending on the severity, you may want to wrap your thigh with a six-inch ace bandage to provide a soft squeeze for support, but not too tight. Only stretch for preventative reasons once the hamstring pain is better.

Once your hamstring pain has subsided, it is recommended that you do leg curls to strengthen the hamstrings. Equally lift one leg at a time so that a strong leg cannot compensate for a weak leg. Also, be sure you focus on engaging your hamstring and not your buttocks or calf.

PROBLEMS WITH OVER-PRONATION

The opposite of supination is over-pronation. Over-pronation in running means excessive inward roll of the foot after landing, such that the foot continues to roll when it should be pushing off. Meaning, those who struggle with over-pronation have a landing whereby their foot rolls inward. Knock knees or flat feet contribute to over-pronation which twists the foot, shin, and knee, causing pain in all those areas. If you are an over-pronator, you will find excessive wear on the inner side of your running shoes, and they will tilt inward if you place them on a flat surface.

Again, shoe technology can help. It is recommended that over-pronators wear shoes with straight or semi-curved soles. The best option are motion control or stability shoes with firm, multi-density midsoles and external control features that limit pronation. Over the counter orthotics or arch supports are also very helpful.

You can tell whether you are making improvements to your over-pronation tendencies by observing the wear pattern on your shoes. The goal is to have "normal" wear and tear on your shoe bottom with an even amount of wear all around.

RECOVERING FROM STRESS FRACTURES

Unfortunately, runners do develop stress fractures while running and training for races. A stress fracture is a fatigued fracture similar to what occurs in metal when it is bent too many times at a specific point. Questions arise what the recovery is like until you are able to run again. Stress fractures are serious and can be recurrent among distance runners, normally taking six to eight weeks to heal. There must be no running during this recovery period.

Furthermore, if you're getting adequate calcium and rest, the stress fracture response may produce a stronger bone. A good plan while recovering is to cross-train. Water running or stationary cycling is a good start with your rehab, and it's recommended you come back slowly with three to four months of easy running. Keep in mind early on in its symptoms, stress fractures may not show up on an X-ray but if you suspect the worse then order an MRI, and if you have a fracture, it will unfortunately show. However, the earlier one can determine this type of diagnosis the faster you will get back to running after appropriate rest.

Remember to be cautious during this recovery period and be sensitive to any foot pain you get during this time. Be sure not to ignore any bone or joint pains as these can be signs of returning trouble. Athletes are advised the minimum amount of time to wait before running a marathon distance is nine months and if your pain returns during this period, go back and see a specialist.

CAUSES OF HEEL PAIN

Heel pain is most often caused by plantar fasciitis, which is a common problem that is related to injury or overuse of the band of tissue attached to the heel. This band of tissue called the plantar fascia is a threadlike tissue that runs the length of the arch, from the heel bone to the toes. The fascia is not very stretchable and that is where your heel problems can begin. Any movement that repeatedly puts too much stretch on the arch and on the plantar fascia can cause the fascia to become inflamed.

Chronic strain of this tissue may lead to formation of a "heel spur." Heel spurs are growths of calcium on the underside of the heel bone. This condition is commonly blamed for the pain you feel, but the pain is actually the result of chronic strain on the plantar fascia and not the spur. If your pain is concentrated in front of the heel pad and is worse in the morning when rising or after a long rest, then you probably have plantar fasciitis. It's rather common that athletes at some point will experience heel pain. The causes of heel pain are varied so the most common causes are as follows:

1. Shoes that do not support the foot.

2. Walking on hard floors.

3. Foot injury.

4. Flat pronated feet.

5. High arched rigid feet.

6. Sudden increase in activity level.

7. Standing on a hard floor for a long time.

8. Obesity.

9. Any movement that repeatedly stretches the plantar fascia.

WHAT CAN YOU DO FOR HEEL PAIN?

Heel pain usually responds slowly to treatment and often requires a variety of treatment options so provided are several solutions:

1. Give your foot a rest for two to six weeks and skip activities such as running, walking, tennis, jumping, and other sports until your condition improves. Swimming or biking are exercises that will not make your plantar fasciitis worse.

2. Try nonprescription arch supports which can often be found at shoe sporting stores and drug stores.

3. Massage the painful area with ice for ten minutes two to three times per day. Do not apply heat.

4. Wear shoes with good arch support and heel support.

5. Stretch your Achilles tendon:
   - Stand at arm's length from the wall or counter with your back knee locked straight and your front knee bent.
   - Your toes should point in slightly.
   - Slowly lean forward until a moderate stretch is felt on your calf muscle of your straight leg.
   - Hold twenty seconds keeping your feet and heels flat on the floor. Do not bounce.
   - Repeat these three to five times on each leg, four times per day.
   - Another stretch with the Achilles tendon is to wrap a towel around the ball of your foot and, keeping your leg straight, gently pull the ball of your foot towards you and hold ten to twenty seconds. Repeat this stretch ten times on each foot.
   - There are two ways to stretch the Achilles tendon in bed:

- o Before getting out of bed wrap a towel around the ball of your foot.
- o Keeping your leg straight, gently pull the ball of your foot towards you and hold ten to twenty seconds.
- Repeat this stretch ten times on each foot.

Try wearing running or walking shoes. Do not walk barefoot. In particular, for women, shoes with a small heel (1 to 1 ½ inches) can also help take some stress off the plantar fascia and provide relief for this condition. Shoes should have a firm heel counter, which is the leather that surrounds the sides and back of the heel.

Finally, give your foot a rest from running until your condition improves. Swimming or biking are excellent alternative exercises that will not make your plantar fasciitis worse.

LOOSE TOES, HAPPY FASCIITIS

As discussed, plantar fasciitis is inflammation of the ligament that runs underneath your foot from the sole to the heel. It's caused by overuse. Consider how much we require of our fasciitis. This sturdy and reliable band of tissue takes on a big responsibility! It supports our every step and is bound to get wound up and tight eventually. Our fasciitis needs a little TLC to continue to support our active lifestyle.

While plantar fasciitis isn't really a toe problem, stretches involving your toes can help prevent and relieve it. Shown below are a few recommended toes stretches.

Toe extension - You should feel this stretch under your foot. Massage the arch of your foot with your thumbs while doing this stretch to increase its effectiveness.

- Sit with your feet flat on the floor.
- Lift the leg with the sore foot and place that ankle on the opposite leg.
- Flex your toes up toward your shin.
- Hold for 5 seconds.
- Relax your toes.
- Repeat 10 times.

Bottle roll - While rolling the bottle, focus on painful areas on the bottom of your foot.

- Sit with your feet flat on the floor.
- Place a bottle of frozen water on the floor in front of you.
- Place the sore foot on the bottle.
- Roll the bottle around with your foot.
- Continue for 1 to 2 minutes.

Ball roll – While rolling the ball, focus on painful areas on the bottom of your foot.

- Sit with your feet flat on the floor.
- Place a golf or tennis ball on the floor in front of you.
- Place the sore foot on the ball.
- Roll the bottle around with your foot.
- Continue for 1 to 2 minutes.

HOW TO ICE AN INJURY?

Ice is one of an athlete's best friends. It is an especially effective treatment for most of the injuries that runners experience. Ice alleviates muscle strain and spasms, prevents hemorrhaging, and reduces swelling of many injuries. Using ice improperly actually can aggravate an injury or cause frostbite. Applying ice for too long a time can cause increased swelling and bleeding. Furthermore, cold increases the permeability of the lymphatic vessels that carry excess tissue fluids back to the cardiovascular system. If an area is iced too long, greater swelling and pain may result.

Apply ice to an injury for twenty minutes followed by a thirty-minute break and then followed by another twenty minutes of icing. This procedure can be repeated as often as possible for the first twenty-four to forty-eight hours following an injury, then three to five times a day until the injury is healed. Heat can be alternated with icing after forty-eight hours. It's recommended to never use heat immediately after an injury. This will cause increased swelling and pain to the injured area. Heat does not have the anti-inflammatory effect that ice does, but hot tubs and heating pads can be very relaxing to your muscles and your mind. Go ahead and use them if you want but rubs and balms applied to the skin have no healing effect. They create a mild stinging sensation in the skin to trick the brain and distract you from your pain.

A more common effective way to ice an injury is to cover the skin with two layers of plastic wrap, Ace bandage, or tight-fitting clothing such as spandex. Once could effectively ice another way by icing for twenty minutes, stop for ten, ice for twenty, stop for ten. If you can do three times a day for three days in a row you get tremendous anti-inflammatory effect. If you don't have the time for this regimen, do what you can. Crushed ice, one-to-two-pound bags of frozen peas, and gel packs work great too.

GENERAL GUIDELINES FOR AVOIDING ACHES FROM RUNNING

At some point in one's running career, it's inevitable aches and pains will occur so recommended below are some of the guidelines to prevent these potential problems. Proper stretching increases the range of motion of your muscles and reduces the chances of being injured and improves your level of performance.

Avoid doing too much running too soon. A guideline is to limit any increase in your weekly running distance to just 10 percent or less of your previous week's total. Try to incorporate an easy week into your running program so, for example, every four weeks, run one week relatively easy. Always follow a hard day of running with an easier day or two. Treat all injuries immediately and properly and see a sports medicine specialist if your pain does not respond to self-treatment. Replace your running shoes every 300 miles and listen to your body and don't exercise too much too quickly. It's recommended you incorporate once a week active recovery (cross-training) like cycling or swimming.

LEARN TO SPOT AN OVERUSE INJURY

There are many activities that stress repetitive movements such as aerobics, cycling, swimming, and running. Unfortunately, these types of fitness pursuits tend to cause overuse injuries. There are many reasons why you can develop such an injury. Outlined below are five reasons why overuse injuries occur:

Inadequate conditioning: When you increase your workload before you are ready to progress you can overstress your body.

Improper technique: Some runners seem to float along in a natural way while others run awkwardly. If you are the latter, learn proper form and technique.

Generic configuration of your body: The way you are built will affect your athletic performance. For example, if you are knock-kneed with wide hips and you take up running, you could develop problems in your knees.

Improper equipment: The way your shoes fit can set up for injury. This includes shoes that are lacking adequate cushioning or arch and heel support.

Type of exercise: Running is more likely to cause overuse injuries of the lower extremities and the back than other sports. In contrast, tennis players are likely to have more shoulder and elbow pain. Listen to your body.

COMMON OVERUSE INJURIES

Almost any muscle, bone, tendon, or joint in your body can become inflamed if you use it improperly and too often. Below is a list of some of the more common overuse injuries.

Shin splints is a broad term for pain that shows up in the front part of the lower leg. The muscles that flex your ankles become sore from overuse and may tear away slightly from the bone. This condition most often results from a combination of weak shin muscles and doing too much too quickly in a running program. Other factors may contribute, including too-tight Achilles tendons, running on a hard surface, or inadequate cushioning in the shoes. Sometimes it's just a matter of wearing a new pair of shoes that will cure shin splints so if you have been running in your current shoes for over 300 miles this would be an ideal opportunity to purchase a new pair.

Shinbone pain on the inner border of the bone, just above the ankle, is usually caused by stretching of the posterior tibia muscle. To prevent this injury or to rectify it early, use shoe inserts that provide extra arch support. You can also do heel raises and other exercises that will strengthen the posterior tibia muscle.

Compartment syndrome is a condition caused by inflammation of the muscles on the front or the outside of the shin. The muscles swell and put pressure on the nerves and blood vessels in the foot and ankle. This condition must be treated immediately.

Stress fractures are tiny, painful cracks that come from repeated stress on bones. They occur in the lower leg, foot, and hip with runners. Stress fractures are often difficult to diagnose and bone scans or other X-ray studies may be necessary. In fact, most experts would recommend that stress fractures may not show up on the X-ray until three weeks after experiencing this condition. An MRI (magnetic resonance imaging) is considered the best way to diagnose stress fractures and can visualize lower grade stress injuries before an X-ray shows changes. Rest from running will allow the fracture to heal itself. With this condition you can substitute another exercise that doesn't put stress on that particular bone.

Achilles tendinitis starts with pain just an inch or two above the heel bone. This is another condition that is best treated by substituting a different exercise, although sometimes a heel lift in your shoe can help as it keeps the tendon from stretching too far.

Bursitis is inflammation of a fluid-filled sac that serves to lubricate areas where the bones and tendons rub together. It is brought about by constant repetitive motion, and runners are prone to bursitis of the knees and hips.

Knowledge is power and the more you are aware of the common types of injuries the better chance you will prevent them from occurring.

VIGOROUS EXERCISE CAN LEAD TO GI SYMPTOMS

According to IFFGD, a nonprofit education and research organization whose mission is to inform, assist and support people affected by gastrointestinal disorders, there is evidence that exercise can contribute to GI disorders including diarrhea and gastroesophageal reflux. It's believed by experts that intense exercise leads to GI symptoms, and untreated reflux which causes heartburn is common. Most often reflux happens when the muscle between the esophagus and the stomach relaxes at the wrong time. Evidence now supports the notion the type of exercise one is involved with can affect reflux episodes. The high impact effects of running appear to cause more reflux episodes than a similar workload involving a low impact exercise like cycling.

Diarrhea and needing a bathroom within minutes after feeling the urge to have a bowel movement are common symptoms found in long-distance runners, especially those running marathons. Research has shown that a marked drop in the blood flow to the colon and small bowel occurs during episodes of extreme exertion. Whether further evaluation and medical treatment in an athlete experiencing diarrhea is called for depends on a number of factors including the person's age and severity of symptoms. It goes on to share that bleeding and persistent diarrhea may signal a severe condition and should always be brought to the attention of a doctor. Mild occasional symptoms should respond to altering the exercise routine and reducing the level of exertion.

Reference: *"Can Intense Exercise Lead to GI Symptoms."* By Renata Korczak, RD CSSD, Teaching Assistant Professor, University of Minnesota; adapted from an article by Thomas Puetz, M.D., Department of Gastroenterology, Aurora Advanced Healthcare, Mequon, WI. Edited by William D. Chey, MD, AGAF, FACG, FACP, RFF Nostrant Collegiate Professor, University of Michigan, Ann Arbor, MI International Foundation for Gastrointestinal Disorders (www.iffgd.org).

APPROACHING SOMEONE WITH AN EATING DISORDER

Unfortunately, there are many people who suffer from eating disorders. If you discover someone that you suspect has an eating disorder, what should you do? Those who suffer from this disorder are reluctant to have a conversation about it for fear of judgement. Naturally, this is a very private topic.

Resolving issues like this should be left to professionals; however, if you are concerned about a friend, you may simply tell them that you are worried about his/her health. One approach is to mention that they seem unhappy or tired, or that you have noticed they don't have the energy to finish workouts, or that they aren't healing from an injury as quickly as expected. Reinforce that you just want them to be happy and healthy. Avoid talking about food and weight since they will likely shut down if you mention anything along those lines.

Don't expect people with an eating disorder to immediately open up to you. It takes time. That said, this disorder can be life-threatening, so if someone you know is really struggling, then you should help them get professional support.

CHRONICALLY FATIGUED ATHLETES

Chronically fatigued athletes commonly take pride in the fact that they haven't missed a day of training in years. They overlook the fact that one or two rest days per week can allow the muscles time to replenish their depleted muscle glycogen. If you have trouble taking a rest day or an easy day, you might want to evaluate whether you are a compulsive exerciser punishing your body or a serious athlete training wisely and improving consistently.

Chronic fatigue can also be a symptom of a medical problem that may be unrelated to nutrition and deserves attention from a physician. However, many complaints can be resolved with better eating, sleeping, and training habits. If you suspect that inappropriate nutrition contributes to your fatigue, you may want to consult a registered dietician or a sports nutritionist.

WHEN YOU EXERCISE REGULARLY, WHY DOESN'T ONE LOSE WEIGHT?

To lose weight, you have to burn off more calories than you eat. Some people do this by adding exercise. In the process, they lose fat but build muscle and weigh the same. Other people exercise but end up eating more. Even though they eat fat-free foods, they get plenty of calories that negate the deficit. Due to fat creating a feeling of fullness, people who eliminate fat often tend to feel hungry and continue to eat. Those calories add up!

You might have better success if you include only a small amount of fat with each meal. For example, most female athletes can lose weight on about 1,600 to 1,800 calories per day. Given that 25 percent of calories can appropriately come from fat, they can eat thirty-five to fifty grams of fat per day.

WHEN TO SEEK ASSISTANCE IF YOU ARE SUFFERING FROM DEPRESSION

Depression can affect people from different backgrounds and runners are not immune to this. Are you feeling sad or tired? Does everything seem overwhelming? Even though exercise can help if you are feeling sad, the fact remains you may be suffering from depression. There are symptoms to look for, so provided are seven of them:

1. Feeling of worthlessness or guilt
2. Changes in sleep pattern
3. Lack of pleasure from usual activities
4. Changes in appetite and weight
5. Restlessness or irritability
6. Difficulty thinking, concentrating, and making decisions
7. Lack of enthusiasm

If you have experienced five or more of the above symptoms for longer than two weeks or your symptoms are interfering with your daily routines, then it's recommended you need to contact your doctor. Recognizing the symptoms and asking for assistance is the first and most important step toward feeling better. Most likely your doctor will determine the most appropriate treatment for you. Keep in mind one out of eight men and one out of four women suffer from depression at some point in their lives. Furthermore, 75% of American college students suffer one time or another from mild depression during their four-year college career.

BEING IMPACTED BY THE FLU

The flu is an infection of the nose, throat, and lungs that is caused by the influenza virus. It occurs every year mainly in late fall and early winter. The flu is an illness of the respiratory system. Most people with the flu feel tired and have a fever, headache, dry cough, sore throat, runny or stuffy nose, sore muscles, and generalized weakness. About 10 to 20 percent of people in the United States get the flu every year and more than 200,000 are admitted to a hospital for complications related to the flu. Each year roughly 20,000 Americans die from these complications. Most of these deaths occur in those older than sixty-five years.

The flu can be spread from person to person. People who have the flu usually cough, sneeze, and have a runny nose. This makes droplets with virus in them, and other people can get the flu by breathing in these droplets. To feel better when you are sick, so you can safely get back to your training, follow the seven recommendations I have listed below:

1. Drink plenty of fluids.

2. Get plenty of rest.

3. Use medicine that reduces fever when needed.

4. Prevent infections by washing hands thoroughly.

5. Keep immunizations up to date, especially for the flu and pneumonia.

6. Use a humidifier or breathe moist air.

7. Use saline nose spray to ease dry nasal passages.

There are times when having the flu can actually sideline you longer than a minor injury so it's important to protect your immune system.

HOW CAN I PROTECT MYSELF FROM THE FLU?

When the flu season breaks out, experts recommend a flu vaccine is the best way to protect against the flu. The viruses in the vaccine change each year based on international surveillance about what types and strains of viruses will circulate in a given year. Approximately two weeks after vaccination, antibodies that provide protection against influenza virus infection develop in the body.

There are also anti-viral drugs that can treat the flu or prevent infection with flu viruses. For treatment, antiviral drugs should be started within forty-eight hours of getting sick. These drugs must be prescribed by a medical professional. It's recommended to athletes to cover your nose and mouth with a tissue when you cough or sneeze. Furthermore, wash your hands often with soap and water, especially after you cough or sneeze. If you don't have access to soap and water at the time you need it, then rubbing your hands together is a secondary option. It's always wise to limit your contact with people who are sick.

INFORMATION ABOUT ENLARGED HEART

An enlarged heart is a sign that the heart is overworked, and heart enlargement can be pathological, which is related to significant heart disease, or physiological related to exercise. An enlarged heart is an indication of an underlying condition. If it's associated with heart disease, doctors will often attempt to treat the underlying disease at the same time as the enlarged heart.

An enlarged heart is often present during heart failure when the heart cannot pump adequate blood to meet the metabolic needs of the body. An enlarged heart may cause symptoms such as shortness of breath, dizziness, or irregular heartbeat. Treatment for an enlarged heart can include medications like beta blockers and controlling other conditions such as high blood pressure. With proper treatment the condition may be controlled or even reversed.

SHOULD ELITE RUNNERS PARTICIPATE IN MORE REGULAR COMPREHENSIVE HEART SCREENINGS?

Many elite athletes have hearts that grow enlarged from training. In rare cases, sudden death can result if the walls of the heart grow thicker than normal, and it becomes fatally difficult for the muscle to pump blood. Perhaps it's time to encourage elite runners to get more regular and comprehensive health screenings. It's a fact that marathoners often sustain heart rates over 180 for more than two hours of racing. Much of the testing they undergo now is to measure race fitness more than overall health. Athletes having sudden death occurs very rarely.

Reference: www.cardiachealth.org/palpitations/sudden-death-in-athletes/

STEPS TO REDUCE THE HEALTH HAZARDS OF SMOKE

Simple measures can go a long way to reduce exposure to wildfire particulate matter. These fires produce obvious health hazards when you can see the smoke, but even air that looks clear can contain particles that are dangerous, which is why you don't exercise outdoors and keep doors closed. Pay attention to symptoms and take precautions such as exercising indoors for a period of time after the fire is out. Those living in the wildfire zones are wise to take precautions for two weeks depending on how quickly the smoke dissipates.

Fire-related symptoms include coughing, shortness of breath, wheezing, and chest pain. If you have any of these symptoms, see a doctor as soon as possible. There are some symptoms that may show up after the fires so do not ignore them. If you must go outdoors and it's smoky, wear a dust mask or hold a wet towel over your face. When indoors keep on the air conditioning if it's smoky outside.

HYPERTENSION RISK FACTORS

The following risk factors for hypertension include age, race, heredity, sex, obesity, stress, smoking, lack of exercise, and diabetes.

Age: High blood pressure is more likely in men over age thirty-five and in women over age forty-five.

Race: Statistically, African Americans are more likely to develop hypertension than Caucasians, and Hispanics also develop hypertension more often than Caucasians.

Heredity: Hypertension runs in some families. A person is 45 percent more likely to have high blood pressure if both parents have it; 28 percent if one parent has it; and 30 percent if one sibling is affected. When one person has hypertension, everyone in the family should have their blood pressure checked regularly.

Sex: Men are more likely to have high blood pressure than women until women become menopausal, when the rate of hypertension exceeds that of men.

Obesity: For every ten pounds of weight gain, blood pressure goes up three to four points. Blood pressure drops when a person loses weight.

Stress: Stress raises heart rate and blood pressure, increasing the workload on the heart. People under stress develop more cardiovascular diseases compared to those who are able to manage stress in their lives.

Smoking: Cigarette smoking significantly increases the risk of hypertension and blood pressure-related illnesses leading to sudden death. Smoking is the highest risk factor for heart disease.

Lack of Exercise: Inactivity leads to weight gain and reduced circulation. Exercise helps to strengthen the blood vessels and reduce blood pressure.

Diabetes: Approximately half of all diabetics develop hypertension. When a diabetic has high blood pressure, their risk of heart attack, stroke, kidney failure, and blindness all increase.

THE SERIOUS THREAT OF HYPERTENSION

Approximately 60 million Americans are estimated to have high blood pressure, or hypertension. Hypertension is defined as a condition in which the force of blood pushing against the walls of the blood vessels is increased. This condition can be mild, moderate, or severe. The specific cause of hypertension is unknown in 90 percent of people but certain risk factors occur.

It is very important to control blood pressure because of the serious threat that it presents to one's health. This condition is often referred to as the silent killer. For example, strokes can result from uncontrolled, severe hypertension. Congestive heart failure can result due to longstanding hypertension. Blood clots can get lodged in narrow arteries that occur when the blood pressure is very high, and this can block the flow of blood resulting in heart attacks and strokes.

People who once thought their blood pressure was fine actually need to start exercising and eating better. While doctors do not usually worry about a patient's blood pressure until it reaches 140/90, the new guidelines say the higher the blood pressure, the greater the chance of these heart diseases. It's estimated that high blood pressure or hypertension affects about a billion people worldwide.

In the United States only about 34 percent of people with high blood pressure have it under control. Blood pressure is measured by two numbers with the top number, systolic blood pressure, referring to the pressure of blood in the arteries when the heart muscle contracts, sending blood to the rest of the body. The bottom number is diastolic blood pressure which refers to the pressure of blood on the arteries when the heart muscle relaxes. It was once believed that the lower diastolic number in a blood pressure reading was the more important reading, but it's now believed that in men and women older than fifty the top systolic number is in fact more likely to predict heart disease. A normal blood pressure reading is 110/70.

HIGH-RISK PREGNANCIES

Healthy women who have a low-risk pregnancy can benefit from exercise, which includes controlling unhealthy weight gain, reducing fatigue, and possibly helping with having a short and smooth labor. Researchers continue to examine whether babies born to active mothers experience long-term benefits as opposed to sedentary mothers, but the data is unclear. However, no evidence suggests exercise during pregnancy disadvantages offspring. That said, all women should consult with their doctor about the safety of exercise during their pregnancy since all pregnancies are different. Generally, women who have high-risk pregnancies should avoid exercise. This includes women with pregnancy-induced hypertension, poorly controlled Type One diabetes, and women experiencing persistent second or third trimester bleeding. Women with cardiovascular, pulmonary, or metabolic disease should be monitored by a doctor during pregnancy. When teaching Health and Lifestyle at San Diego City College and discussing the chapter on prenatal care, I often stress the importance that women who exercise while pregnant should monitor their body's reaction for unusual symptoms. The following are signs that signal to stop exercise and consult a doctor:

- Vaginal bleeding
- Loss of amniotic fluid
- Unusual shortness of breath
- Dizziness or severe headaches
- Chest pain
- Muscle weakness
- Painful uterine contractions

The good news is these are very rare occurrences and women with healthy pregnancies can typically exercise the full term without complications. The type of exercise includes anything that your body is used to, including running.

RECOMMENDED GUIDELINES FOR EXERCISING DURING PREGNANCY

According to the American College of Sports Medicine, the healthiest pregnant women would benefit from at least thirty minutes of moderate activity on most but not all days of the week.

Most women who were active before pregnancy, and especially if they ran, should continue to exercise. The type and intensity of exercise should be based on previous history, health, and comfort. It's recommended that early in a pregnancy, many women can continue to train at moderate intensities. As the pregnancy continues, running exercise intensity usually decreases naturally, and the type, duration and intensity of exercise are sometimes modified with comfort and safety in mind. Keep in mind the baby's heart rate can be ten beats higher than the mother's when she exercises.

According to the American College of Sports Medicine (ACSM), the following important safety concerns should be followed when exercising during pregnancy:

1. Avoid exercise for extended periods in a supine position after the first trimester.

2. Take steps to avoid heat injury.

3. Avoid extremes in barometric pressure, so avoid scuba diving and exercising at altitudes of more than 6,000 feet.

4. Limit the possibility of falling and impact injury.

Sedentary women who are not used to exercising before being pregnant should consult with their doctors. These women can safely engage in low-intensity exercise and for these women, walking is typically recommended for exercise and should be done at moderate speeds.

Reference: ACSM Pregnancy Physical Activity.
https://www.acsm.org/docs/default-source/files-for-resource-library/pregnancy-physical-activity.pdf

THE USE OF STEROIDS HAS SERIOUS NEGATIVE SIDE EFFECTS

Personally, I never used performance-enhancing drugs during my competitive career, but I suspected there were fellow competitors who undoubtedly used and abused drugs to gain advantage over other athletes. Anabolic steroids, a synthetic form of the male hormone testosterone, offer another shortcut. Steroids enhance protein synthesis, thereby producing more rapid and dramatic increases in muscular size and strength. When combined with a strength training program there is no question that steroids do stimulate muscular growth and development.

Due to the very serious negative side effects, the use of steroids has been banned by the Olympic Committee, the NCAA, and other reputable athletic organizations. Steroids do have some legitimate medical value in the treatment of certain blood diseases, growth disorders, breast cancer, asthma, and arthritis. However, prescribing steroids for the purpose of enhancing muscular development, even when done by a medical doctor, is illegal in the US. Unfortunately, steroid use continues to be relatively common among professional, college, and high school athletes. The National Institute on Drug Abuse estimates that as many as 400,000 teenagers are using steroids. The distribution of illegal steroids has become a $500 million operation.

Today's news is filled with stories of notable athletes who are under allegations for using anabolic steroids. The use of steroids has very serious and often permanent physiological and psychological side effects that have been well documented. Steroid use has been shown to increase aggressiveness and contribute to violent outbursts and temper tantrums. Other negative side effects for males include baldness, upper body acne, enlarged breasts, stunted bone development in adolescents, damage to the liver, and enlarged prostate.

Since the testosterone the body needs is being supplied artificially, the function of the testicles is precluded, and shrunken testicles and impotency may result. Steroid use also dramatically increases total cholesterol, decreases HDL, increases LDL, and increases triglycerides. When used by women, steroids lead to masculine traits such as a lower voice, facial hair, cessation of menstrual cycle, and the other negative side effects listed for men. Human growth hormones represent another substance that has been used to enhance muscular size and strength and like steroids, they too have many serious side effects. Finally, the rapid and short-term gains in muscle size and strength by using steroids are limited compared to the negative side effects that can be permanent and potentially life-threatening.

Reference: orthoinfo.aaos.org/en/staying-healthy/the-risks-of-using-performance-enhancing-drugs-in-sports/

SYMPTOMS AND REMEDIES TO HEAT EXHAUSTION AND HEATSTROKE

While in college at San Diego State, the team would head up to Sequoia National Park in August for training camp prior to the upcoming cross-country season. On one extremely hot and muggy day, I got lost on a run and was out in the elements for much longer than expected. As a result, I suffered from heat exhaustion due to excessive loss of water and salt depletion. Symptoms of heat exhaustion include thirst, headache, a pale appearance, dizziness, and possibly nausea or vomiting. In severe cases, your heart will race, and you may feel disoriented.

Heat exhaustion is the precursor to heatstroke. Heatstroke happens when the body's thermoregulatory system stops working. Heatstroke can appear similar to heat exhaustion but is much more severe. Symptoms of heatstroke include cessation of sweating, difficulty walking, disorientation, fainting, or unconsciousness. Runners suffering from heatstroke will be too disoriented to help themselves. It is important to learn to recognize the symptoms of both heat exhaustion and heatstroke and understand they are similar but not the same.

If you or someone you are with experiences heat exhaustion, stop running and get out of the sun and go into an air-conditioned building if possible. Avoid the urge to quickly gulp down water or a sports drink. Rather, drink slowly to allow the liquid to absorb and not bloat your stomach, which can cause vomiting. If you don't improve within thirty minutes, go to the emergency room as soon as possible.

While heat exhaustion is not fatal if treated quickly, heatstroke can be. The key symptom to look for is disorientation. If someone is not mentally functioning well, then they are in danger. Quickly pack ice around the runner's neck, armpit, and groin and splash as much water on the skin as possible. Elevate the legs and if the person is conscious, give them plenty of fluids. One to two quarts of a sports drink is recommended, but water will also work. The person will likely be nauseated and not want to drink anything, but fluids are essential so don't give up! Proceed to call 911 to get the runner to the hospital before it is too late.

IS THERE ANYTHING YOU CAN DO FOR EXERCISE-INDUCED ORGASMS?

Early in my coaching career with the San Diego Track Club, I was approached during a Tuesday workout session by one of my elite female athletes claiming that during the first mile interval, she experienced an orgasm. At first, I thought that I misunderstood. Quite honestly, I was a bit dumbfounded and didn't know what to say.

I asked her to try and run another mile interval; however, during the second timed interval she stopped running midway through. And judging by the expression on her face, I could tell that she was completely in shock and visibly upset. Clearly, she was unable to finish her workout that day. I sympathetically consoled her and told her I would conduct some research and follow back up with her on my findings.

I later consulted another female coach colleague of mine who confirmed that this phenomenon is true. What my athlete experienced was an exercise-induced orgasm, also known as "coregasms."

While rare, some women can experience orgasms through exercise. It is a form of Persistent Genital Arousal Disorder (PGAD) that is sparked by exercising the core muscles. PGAD results in spontaneous, persistent, and uncontrollable genital arousal, with or without orgasm or genital engorgement, unrelated to any feelings of sexual desire. As you can imagine, experiencing repeated coregasms can be scary and very frustrating to a female athlete.

Preventing spontaneous exercise-induced orgasms comes down to identifying triggers and avoiding certain activities. The exercises most associated with coregasms are running, ab exercises on captain's chair, weightlifting, cycling, and climbing a rope.

One recommendation I have for athletes who might experience an orgasm while exercising is to record information and then make an appointment with a healthcare provider or doctor. Your healthcare provider can then use this information to assess symptoms and make a diagnosis.

Provided below are some key points you may want to make note of.

- How you felt and what you were doing before it happened.
- Assess any other unusual physical symptoms and/or over the counter drugs or prescription medications. This is especially true if you believe that your symptoms are connected to a prescription or other drug.
- Consider any recent substance use and determine if this prompted this reaction.

Taking notes will help you and your healthcare provider identify patterns and make recommendations to avoid coregasms from happening during future training sessions.

WHAT I'VE LEARNED

COACH PAUL GREER'S FOUR LIFE LESSONS LEARNED FROM "GOING THE DISTANCE"

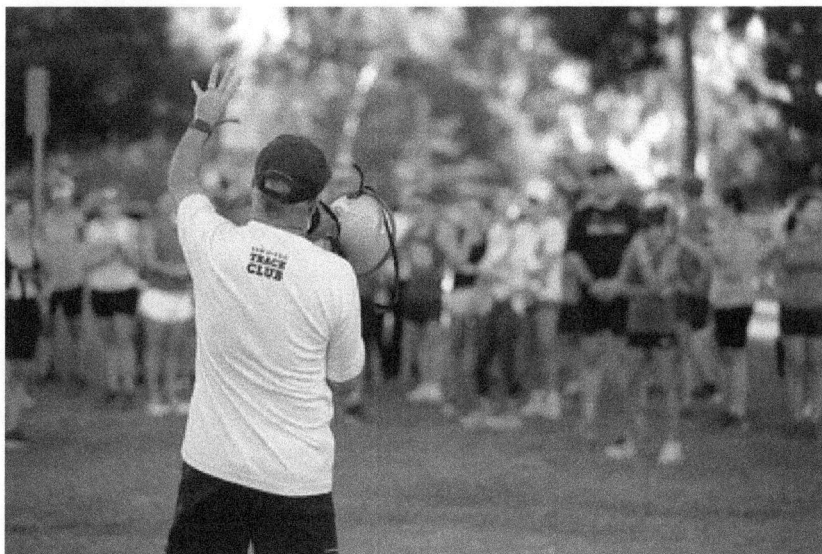

My final tip for this book is now dedicated toward sharing four impactful lessons I have learned from life experiences while working with students and athletes over the years. Personally, I believe these four truths below can provide us all with a sense of peace and happiness as we navigate through this beautiful journey we call life.

Be selfless

One of the greatest definitions of love that I have ever heard came from an immensely influential philosopher, Saint Thomas Aquinas, who stated, *"To love is to will the good of the other."* In other words, one must put others before themselves and do what is best for people who enter our lives regardless of what this means for you — true selflessness. In many ways this is the secret to much of our happiness in life. When we focus our love and attention toward others, life is much more fulfilling. Humanity's greatest

331

limitation is self-centeredness, and we are the least happy and least fulfilled when being obsessed with our own importance.

Tell others they make a difference in your life

A phrase that has resonated with me for years is *"You make a difference in my life."* What started as a simple statement I would shout out during the weekly running workouts, has somehow stuck with me and become my personal mantra. Like it or not, I'm known for this phrase. I constantly and happily repeat this slogan when I teach, when I coach, and any opportunity I get. Thousands of athletes have heard me voice these words through a megaphone (yes, a megaphone) as they arduously hammer through grueling workouts . . . They'll hear me say, *"You all make a difference in my life. Go ahead. Tell the person running next to you that they make a difference."* Sure, some may think it odd that I deliver this message during a workout, but that's me. I joyously spread the word of love and gratitude every opportunity that I get. Every life encounter is an opportunity to share the very best version of yourself so aim at being that instrument of compassion and love.

Learn to forgive

Forgiveness begins from within. Forgiving is accepting others as they are while recognizing one's own underlying anger, prejudices, and imperfections. This is an incredible life challenge; however, the more that you can forgive others while also asking for forgiveness from past transgressions, the more fully you can love and let go of the ignorance, selfishness, greed, and anger from an unforgiving heart. Hold no grudges as they will only drag you down.

The power of giving

There are moments in my own life when I struggle with humility. True humility means putting the needs of another person before your own and thinking of others before yourself. It also means not drawing attention to yourself. You can only be truly happy and self-fulfilled when you are humble and give of yourself for others. Give freely and without inhibition and be filled with true, eternal love.

ABOUT THE AUTHOR

Paul Greer's storied running career began at St. Augustine High School. After being inducted into the school's Hall of Fame in 1995, he went on to become the 1500-meter record-holder at San Diego State University, where his 3:42.44 still stands as the best mark in school history.

Since then, Paul has coached thousands of athletes in endurance sports, including track athletes, marathon runners, Ironman triathletes, and various endurance sport enthusiasts. His students include hundreds of Boston qualifiers, several top age-group competitors, and a handful of Olympic qualifiers.

In addition to his forty years as a coach, Paul is a professor in Health and Exercise Science at San Diego City College, Director for the "Rockin' N Runnin" full and half marathon training program, and a staple of the San Diego running community. His debut book, *Going the Distance: Strategies from the First Stride to the Finish Line*, is the expression of his sincere passion to improve lives through the pursuit of mental and physical excellence.

www.ingramcontent.com/pod-product-compliance
Lightning Source LLC
Chambersburg PA
CBHW032048020426
42335CB00011B/244